HEALING

with CBD

HEALING
with CBD

HOW CANNABIDIOL CAN TRANSFORM
YOUR HEALTH WITHOUT THE HIGH

EILEEN KONIECZNY, RN

with LAUREN WILSON

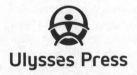

Ulysses Press

Published in the United States by:
Ulysses Press
P.O. Box 3440
Berkeley, CA 94703
www.ulyssespress.com

ISBN: 978-1-61243-829-0
Library of Congress Catalog Number: 2018944071

Printed in Canada by Marquis Book Printing
10 9 8 7 6 5 4 3 2 1

Acquisitions editor: Casie Vogel
Managing editor: Claire Chun
Editor: Renee Rutledge
Proofreader: Shayna Keyles
Front cover design: Rebecca Lown
Interior design and layout: what!design @ whatweb.com
Interior art: page 56, figure outline, Martial Red/shutterstock.com; page 64, Leafly; page 105: plant, PopFoto/shutterstock.com; trichomes, Gleti/shutterstock.com; female flower, NinaM/shutterstock.com; male flower, Hein Nouwens/shutterstock.com; page 190, dropper, vixenkristy/shutterstock.com
Production: Jake Flaherty, Claire Sielaff

Distributed by Publishers Group West

Contents

CHAPTER 9: USING CBD: NOT ONE SIZE FITS ALL 162

CHAPTER 10: HOW MUCH SHOULD I TAKE? 185

Chapter 11: Finding Products You Can Trust.......197

Conclusion.......234

Appendix.......235

Acknowledgments.......267

About the Authors.......269

Introduction

It was years ago now, but I will never forget the day I learned that cannabis can be medicine. I was speaking with a beekeeper friend of mine. He had asked about the health of my sister, who at that time had been living with stage IV breast cancer for the past five years. We spoke about her current chemotherapy regimen, the tingling in her hands, imbalance, fatigue, and the fog they call chemo-brain.

He asked me if she ever used cannabis, and I was surprised by the question. Having a brother who had issues with drugs and alcohol, cannabis did not factor positively in my life. My friend began to tell me about the history of the plant and how safe it was, how it was used as medicine "back in the day." He called it a "truly amazing plant" and that he knew people who used it to help tolerate their chemotherapy. It was that conversation that changed the path of my life, and I have never looked back.

My name is Eileen Konieczny, and I have been a registered nurse for over 25 years. My specialty is bedside nursing care for patients diagnosed with cancer. I have run the gamut within oncology: oncology nursing certification, stem cell transplants, high dose chemotherapy, symptom management, and end of life care.

I am proud of the work I have done as a nurse. Some of the main responsibilities of our profession are to promote and restore health, to prevent illness, and to alleviate the suffering of individuals and society at large. This is done respectfully and unrestricted by considerations of age, color, creed, culture, disability or illness, gender, sexual orientation, nationality, politics, race, or social status. Everyone looks the same in a hospital gown and it has been my greatest honor to be of service to people when they are experiencing some of the darkest times of their lives. It certainly isn't for everyone, but like with many of my colleagues, it is a calling.

So it is with the education and experience of a nurse and the heart of a daughter and sister that I began my journey to understand cannabis as medicine. This book is a step forward in this journey.

My Journey

My mom was diagnosed with pancreatic cancer the month after my wedding, January 1996. She had died by the end of that summer. I watched her shrink to mere skin and bones before my eyes. She had no desire for food; nothing had enough taste to waste energy eating. Oh, how she wanted food to taste like food again.

Had I known or thought to consider cannabis then, I believe she would have tried it. And knowing the value of utilizing cannabinoids for health and wellness, I believe she would have experienced a better end to her life. I believe she would have eaten more, laughed more, and experienced less pain.

For the past ten years, I have educated myself and anyone else who would listen about the medicinal benefits of cannabis. The more I learned, the louder I became. I remember many of the patients I cared for over the years and the limitations I faced trying to alleviate their suffering.

I remember what was lacking in the care of my mother and sister.

I have vivid memories of a trip I took with my sister to California. She was diagnosed with metastatic breast cancer within a year of giving birth to my niece, and I was painfully aware of what the years ahead of her would hold. In the later years of her diagnosis, the breast cancer cells that had already been in her liver also went into her brain. This made traveling alone dangerous of her, so when I announced that I would be traveling to California for a seminar on cannabis, I was surprised when she decided to come along.

Traveling together had always been a joy, filled with plenty of laughs, beautiful scenery, and great company. Unfortunately, early on in this trip she insisted that I stop talking about pot. I was deeply entrenched in my cannabis education and had an irritating habit of preaching about the incredible things I was learning, making it *the* topic of conversation most of the time we were together. My sister had no interest in using cannabis in any form. She didn't care about the information that I was learning, that I was desperate for her to hear.

So I stopped talking about it and our days became very quiet. She never did try using cannabis.

My memory often takes me back to get glimpses of significant moments in my life, and that trip is one of them. It had lasting effects for me—on a personal level, I have learned to temper my enthusiasm and be mindful of the boundaries of others. On a professional level, I quickly became part of a small yet growing number of healthcare professionals who stand up, educate, and advocate for safe access to cannabis medicine.

Here is a plant that has been used safely for thousands of years in traditional and western medicinal practices; anecdotally helps individuals cope with the side effects of chemotherapy, pain, and other maladies; and has research that points to what Raphael Mechoulam, PhD, a pioneer in the field of cannabis research, calls a "treasure trove" of bioactive compounds that are known to have beneficial, therapeutic, and medicinal effects.

If that isn't enough, in the early 1990s, researchers uncovered a newly discovered endocannabinoid system (ECS). The ECS is a system that is inherent and hard-wired within our body, and whose job it is to maintain homeostasis: a balanced internal environment despite the daily fluctuation in our external environment (poor diet, pollution, stress). It does this by continuously regulating functions in our brain, skin, digestive tract, liver, cardiovascular system, genitourinary function, and even bone.

I am keenly aware of the controversies surrounding cannabis, and I choose to fight for safe, legal access to cannabinoid-based medicines and supplements that support wellness and alleviate patient pain and suffering. I feel so strongly about this information and its suppression that I have left bedside hospital nursing for it.

HEALING with CBD

One of the absurdities of cannabis is that it is illegal for any purpose, which we will go into further detail later in this book. But briefly, for context, cannabis and its constituents are designated as a Schedule I drug, which from a legal and regulatory viewpoint means it has a high potential for addiction, no medical value, and cannot be used safely under the supervision of a physician. The use of cannabis as medicine is illegal in states that have not passed legislation that allows for its use.

I was working in Connecticut when I began this journey of cannabis advocacy, which at that time did not have laws permitting the use of medical cannabis. Looking back, my first steps into advocacy included writing letters to my elected officials, asking my nursing colleagues if they were taught about the endocannabinoid system, and asking my patients if they ever considered alternative treatments, taking the conversation to cannabis if they were receptive to the topic.

It became clear that I had overstepped my bounds, according to hospital management, when I was required to sign a document that allowed for my immediate dismissal if I continued to speak to my patients about the use of cannabis as a medicine. Sometimes, what a nurse has in her toolbox is never enough. I remember feeling dismayed for what I considered ignorance on the part of my supervisors. I knew the only way to fix the problem, to allow patients the right to choose a safe alternative, was to make medical cannabis legal.

With so few healthcare professionals interested in cannabis as medicine, I channeled my effort and voice advocating on a state level for patients' rights. I'm honored to have played an integral role in the passage of Connecticut Chapter 420f: The Palliative Use of Marijuana.

With safe access guaranteed to CT residents, I began talking to patients again but was quickly reminded of my gag order. Despite the recent political victory, my hospital (like many others) was conflicted on the disparities between federal and state law, particularly as it received federal monies associated with Medicare. It was then that I knew my experience and strong beliefs were better served elsewhere. Leaving the bedside was a difficult but necessary step along this journey.

Since then I have watched and participated in the growth of an industry. I stepped up and spoke out on behalf of the patients living in my home state, New York, playing an integral role in medical cannabis legislation in 2014. I have also co-founded two companies that produce lab-tested, standardized doses of cannabinoid based medicines, served as President of the American Cannabis Nurses Association, and continue to help thousands of patients navigate the rocky terrain of medicinal cannabis treatment.

With access to medical cannabis spreading across the country and patients and consumers alike becoming increasingly aware of the potential benefits that cannabinoids offer when treating various ailments, the need for unbiased information is at a premium.

As a nurse, one of my responsibilities is to make sure that my patients know where their blind spots are, understanding options that they didn't know about—the stuff they didn't know they didn't know.

Knowledge is empowering. It can help you to feel more "in control" of your condition and the impact it has on your life and that of your family. Thank you for joining us on this journey.

What to Expect from This Book

This book was designed to be a practical, no-fuss guide for using cannabidiol. You can jump right to the information on how to find and use CBD products, then go on your merry way! If and when you would like to dive deeper into the science of cannabis and how it interacts with your body, that information will be there for you, too. And if you're feeling a particular newfound (or long-burning) affinity for the plant and want to learn more about its fascinating history and the social/political context in which it currently exists, we've provided a primer on those topics in Chapters 2 and 3.

At the end of this book, you will find a whole section that contains a solid list of electronic and print resources to help you learn more, because this is a rich and complicated topic and each chapter in this book could be its own book! (And some are, so check out that resource section.) You will also find several **bold** words throughout the book to highlight key definitions, and a glossary at the end of the book as well.

There is really no wrong way to use this book, and we hope it proves to be useful to you on your journey to wellness!

CHAPTER 1

WHAT'S ALL THE BUZZ ABOUT?

"Simply put, and politics aside, marijuana is the single most medicinally valuable plant that has ever existed."
  —Michael H. Moskowitz, MD, in *CBD: A Patient's Guide to Medicinal Cannabis*

If you're reading this book, chances are you already know that cannabidiol (CBD) is the cannabis medicine *du jour*. CBD is being put into everything from sparkling water to deodorant, and consumer enthusiasm for CBD-infused products is at an all-time high.

So why all the buzz? Part of the reason is certainly due to the fact that CBD won't give you a buzz—cannabidiol won't get you high like its cannabinoid cousin tetrahydrocannabinol (THC). But the recent trend toward putting CBD into anything and everything (aside from cashing in on all the hype around CBD among the general public) largely comes from the fact that CBD shows promise in treating a laundry list of conditions longer than your arm—and any psoriasis that might be on that arm, too.

People are often amazed by the touted ability of cannabis to treat a large variety of seemingly unrelated conditions. But we now understand that all of these conditions are regulated, at least in part, by the **endogenous cannabinoid system** (endocannabinoid system, or ECS). The endocannabinoid system is the primary way that cannabidiol, along with all the other beneficial compounds in cannabis and hemp, interacts with your body. It is an innate biological system present in all mammals and other living creatures that bridges many physiological locations and other systems in the body, and impacts bodily functions as basic as eating, sleeping, relaxing, immunity, and memory formation (see Chapter 4: Cannabinoids and The Entourage Effect for more).

The cell receptors that make use of CBD and other cannabinoids are located all over the body, from the deepest primal parts of the brain to the dark recesses of the gut to the surface of the skin. This means that CBD can be consumed in a variety of ways, or through a variety of delivery methods (see How Can I Take CBD? on page 167), which has also influenced the boon in all things CBD-infused.

CBD's effects on our most basic bodily functions while working all over the body at the cellular level means it has the *potential* to help with any number of conditions that severely impact the quality of life of millions of people living with various conditions—Parkinson's, multiple sclerosis (MS), fibromyalgia, and epilepsy, for example. Why the conscious use of the word "potential"? Because the science supporting CBD's therapeutic uses is still in its infancy, and CBD's rise in popularity is relatively new, within the last decade.

In fact, the discovery of the whole endocannabinoid system is a relatively new thing as well. We have only known about the ECS for about 25 years (a very short time frame in the context of medical research). Dr. Raphael Mechoulam, widely regarded as the grandfather of cannabis science, and his colleagues discovered the ECS in the early '90s.

While it may seem like we know a lot about cannabinoids, the estimated twenty thousand scientific articles on the topic have just begun to scratch the surface. Large gaps still exist in our current knowledge around the complexity of interactions that happen in the ECS between various cannabinoids, cell types, and other bodily systems.

While preclinical trials of CBD-based therapies are proving very promising and exciting in a large variety of therapeutic applications, we are still a long way from understanding all the ways in which CBD works in our bodies and how we can use CBD best as a medicine.

CBD Research: Preclinical Studies vs. Clinical Trials

When new medications are being developed, they go through various stages of study and testing before being approved for public consumption, a process that takes many years to complete. Preclinical studies are done before human testing (called "clinical trials") can be carried out, and typically, animal test subjects are used. While positive preclinical test results are encouraging, often medications that test well in animals do not translate as expected in human test subjects. So while we can infer a lot from preclinical studies, we don't have a lot of clinical data to rigorously back up our initial ideas on CBD just yet.

Another complicating factor on the cannabis science front is that research has been greatly stunted here in the United States due to the fact that cannabis is considered a Schedule I drug, or categorized as a drug with the highest potential for abuse, with no accepted medical use (see page 33 for details on Schedule 1 drugs). This means that legal research on cannabis has been extremely limited and more interested in proving cannabis is bad for human health, rather than good. The story behind this goes back nearly 100 years, and is fraught with political propaganda and corporate interests winning out over human interests. But the social tides have been shifting, and one need only watch any of the television ads for FDA-approved drugs to realize that the side effects of cannabis don't hold a candle to the risks of pharmaceutical drugs.

Why Now?

This book is important *right now* for a number of reasons. For starters, consumers need a no-nonsense basic understanding of what CBD is and how to use it, so they can seek out the products that will best serve them. Not all CBD products are created equally! This book will help you understand what questions need to be asked as you start your journey with CBD: questions to ask yourself, bud tenders, growers, producers, and even your doctor. It will help you understand how CBD is extracted, concentrated, and used in the seemingly endless array of products now out there on the market. It will also help you know what to look for on product labels, ingredient lists, and lab test results.

While the science supporting CBD might currently be limited, what's not limited is the number of firsthand accounts from people who have been helped by the medicinal properties of cannabis. It is in large part because of all the *anecdotal evidence* and public support for CBD that the science is being pushed to catch up. You will find stories of patients, practitioners, and producers throughout this book; stories from real people who have been helped or have helped others with the all-natural, nontoxic, therapeutic properties of a pretty phenomenal yet often misunderstood plant. In the age of an American opioid crisis and popping pills for every possible ailment, there are many who could experience real benefit from a natural and nontoxic form of medicine. So this book is important right now because more people than ever before can be helped by CBD and cannabis therapeutics.

WHAT IS ANECDOTAL EVIDENCE?

Anecdotal evidence is evidence based on a person's story of their subjective experience. Many of the sidebars you will find in this book contain anecdotal evidence in the form of patient stories. Anecdotal evidence is given little credence by the medical community because it is not backed up by rigorous and thorough scientific investigation or proof. That being said, it can be quite useful in evaluating new drugs and how patients are responding to them. In the case of medical cannabis in the US, patients and their shared experiences have largely been guiding the ship in product development and scientific research since legitimate scientific research continues to be limited by the Schedule I status of cannabis.

In the bigger picture of the cannabis landscape, this book is important right now because unbeknownst to most folks, the fight for legal cannabis has been going on for decades. A passionate and tireless community of educators and advocates (many of them quoted here in this book and referenced in the resource section at the end of the book) are working to get cannabis into the hands of those who need and want it. Contrary to cliché pop-culture depictions, cannabis legalization isn't a smoke-filled stoner's dream—it's something that is being hard fought for across the country. As of this writing, cannabis and/or CBD is legally available in 48 states: 31 states have medical marijuana programs (in addition to the territories of Guam, Puerto Rico, and the District of Columbia), while 17 have CBD-specific legislation allowing for low-THC hemp-derived forms of CBD.

The Current Social Landscape

By and large, the public supports cannabis legalization. According to a Pew Research Center poll from January 2018, 61% of Americans support cannabis legalization. When it comes to medical cannabis use, that number spikes. A Quinnipiac survey (also from January 2018) reported that nearly all Americans (91%) support legalizing cannabis for medical use. As of this writing, 31 states and three territories have legal medical programs, while 9 states plus DC have legalized cannabis for adult use. And this landscape is continually shifting. As of July 2018, here are the states and territories with medical cannabis programs:

1. Alaska

2. Arizona

3. Arkansas

4. California

5. Colorado

6. Connecticut

7. Delaware	21. New Hampshire
8. Washington, DC	22. New Jersey
9. Florida	23. New Mexico
10. Guam	24. New York
11. Hawaii	25. North Dakota
12. Illinois	26. Ohio
13. Louisiana	27. Oklahoma
14. Maine	28. Oregon
15. Maryland	29. Pennsylvania
16. Massachusetts	30. Puerto Rico
17. Michigan	31. Rhode Island
18. Minnesota	32. Vermont
19. Montana	33. Washington
20. Nevada	34. West Virginia

And yet there continues to be a disconnect between state and federal governments. Cannabis is still illegal at the federal level, being classified along with heroin and cocaine as a Schedule I drug (see Chapter 2: A Brief History of Cannabis for details). The federal government can't ignore the issue of legal cannabis, especially since legal sales in North America were $9 billion in 2017 and are projected to be $21 billion in the US by 2021 (according to BDS Analytics).

So how does the current state of cannabis matter to you as someone who is interested in using CBD? It could mean one of several things. Depending on where you live, you might have

HEALING with CBD

full and legal access to CBD products. If you live in an adult-use state like California, Colorado, or Washington, it could be as easy as walking into your local dispensary and asking the bud tender for help. If you have a qualifying condition, getting a medical card in these states could help save you some money, as sales tax tends to be much higher for adult use versus medical use.

If you live in a state that has a medical program but no adult use, you will need to qualify as a medical patient. This means consulting the specific list of conditions covered under your state's program. Conditions that are covered vary from state to state. If you qualify, you will need to get patient certification from a registered practitioner. Once certified, you will receive your medical card and can visit a dispensary to purchase product.

In the rest of the country, at both the state and federal levels, the legality of CBD is firmly stuck in a legal morass. Some states, like Iowa, Alabama, and North Carolina, (there were 17 at the time of this writing, see CBD-Only States) have CBD-specific laws. This means that they have allowed for low-THC (typically less than 0.3% of dry weight, but this can vary from state to state) industrial hemp-derived forms of CBD for medical consumption but do not have broader medical cannabis programs in place. Most of these states, while allowing CBD consumption for approved conditions, allow only for possession. This means that while you can possess CBD, they do not allow for any infrastructure to supply patients with CBD product. As of July 2018, these are states that do not have a medical cannabis program but allow for low-THC hemp-derived CBD products:

1. Alabama	10. South Carolina
2. Georgia	11. South Dakota
3. Indiana	12. Tennessee
4. Iowa	13. Texas
5. Kentucky	14. Utah
6. Mississippi	15. Virginia
7. Missouri	16. Wisconsin
8. North Carolina	17. Wyoming
9. Oklahoma	

See Chapter 7: Sources of CBD: Cannabis and Hemp for more on CBD-only states.

There are producers of hemp-derived CBD products that ship nationwide. Companies like Palmetto Harmony and Bluegrass Hemp Oil produce domestically grown and entirely hemp-based products that ship to all states. As you will learn, CBD derived from hemp versus cannabis vary in efficacy from person to person. While some people have wonderful success with hemp-derived CBD, others find that whole-plant cannabis extracts work better for them (get the full scoop in Chapters 6 and 7).

CHAPTER 2

A Brief History of Cannabis

"The marijuana story is actually many stories, all woven into one grand epic about a remarkable plant that befriended our ancestors, altered their consciousness, and forever changed the word in which we live."

— Martin Lee, from *Smoke Signals: A Social History of Marijuana—Medical, Recreational and Scientific*

In this chapter you will learn about a plant with a scandalous past, *Cannabis sativa*, that has been relegated to a state of prohibition in the United States for the past 80 years and whose wonders are finally coming back to light.

Throughout history, we see evidence to support the importance of the cannabis plant to the development of societies worldwide. From China to India, Africa to Latin America, and Europe to North America, the cannabis plant has been intertwined with religions, migration, colonialism, and political powers.

The genus *Cannabis L.* includes several closely related species. Both hemp and cannabis fall into the same subspecies, *Cannabis sativa*. However, both plants have evolved to become quite different. What we generally refer to as industrial hemp generally contains less than 1 percent THC and has many practical uses (hence "industrial"), while the plant we refer to as cannabis or marijuana is its psychoactive cousin, containing THC percentages between 13% to 30% (as of the date of this publication). The psychoactivity associated with cannabis can be attributed to the compound THC, a cannabinoid that is found in the sticky resin of the female cannabis plants. This resin is where the plant's medicinal compounds are found; the most well-known cannabinoid had been THC until recently, when CBD entered into the limelight.

What Is THC?

Tetrahydrocannabinol is the psychoactive compound found within the resin glands of the cannabis plant. According to the National Institutes of Health, THC binds to specific receptors in the brain called cannabinoid receptors that are found concentrated in areas associated with thinking, memory, pleasure, coordination, and time perception. The "high" associated with cannabis may produce a variety of effects that lead to an altered sense of time and space, enhanced appetite, impaired short-term memory, feelings of happiness, and occasional drowsiness. In low doses, THC has shown promise for its ability to reduce some pain and muscle spasms, stimulate appetite, and help reduce nausea with a safety profile that pharmaceuticals can't compete with.

Each of these effects vary greatly depending on who is using it, their age, how much they are using, how they are using it, and how often. For more on THC and other cannabinoids, see Chapter 4: Cannabinoids and the Entourage Effect.

The Ancient Origins of Medicinal Cannabis

First human contact with cannabis likely happened about 12,000 years ago in Central Asia. This was the Neolithic Period, the time of a hugely important shift in human culture and survival: the very beginnings of farming. Sustainable agriculture (growing crops) is an invention of modern human civilization, dating back only 10,000 years.

Through history, every part of the cannabis plant has been used by humans. Stems and stalks provided fiber for cloth, rope, cords, paper, building materials, and more; the roots, leaves, and flowers were used medicinally and spiritually; and the seeds, as food, provided essential fatty acids and proteins. Capable of growing most anywhere (some might even say it grows like a weed), cannabis is one of the world's oldest cultivated crops.

The mythic Chinese figure Shen Nung (28th century BCE) was said to have documented his experiments with cannabis and hundreds of other medicinal herbs. Revered as the father of Chinese Medicine, it's believed that his work survived through the millennia and was included in the Chinese pharmacopeia *Pen Ts'ao Ching*, the earliest surviving copies of which were penned in the 1st century CE. These writings have formed the basis of much of traditional Chinese medicine, and it advises hemp tinctures for a number of ailments. In the 2nd century CE, cannabis was being mixed with wine to make a preparation called *ma-fei-san* that was used as an anesthetic for surgery.

By 2,000 BCE, cannabis had traveled to India where it was first embraced by both the Buddhist and Hindu religions. From its spiritual beginnings, its use expanded to treat ailments like dysentery and fever. By 1,500 BCE, cannabis had spread to Persia, Greece, Germany, and France, and in 900 BCE, the Middle Eastern Assyrians were using cannabis in their religious rites. It is believed that European cultivation of cannabis may have started around 800 BCE in Germany. Russia was likely an early adopter as well, but in its colder climates, the medicinal properties of the plants would have been minimal and cannabis was likely used primarily for its fibers.

As a primary ingredient in paper, cannabis took on a new importance during the Renaissance when the introduction of Gutenberg's movable-type printing press started an intellectual revolution. And even though European plants had low levels of THC, the plant was still used as medicine. In 1538, the English naturalist William Turner praised it in his book *A New Herball*. The Italian botanist Pietro Andrea Gregorio Mattioli also wrote about its therapeutic effects around the same time. In 1649, an English herbalist named Nicholas Culpeper collected these accounts in his book *A Physicall Directory*. He discusses uses for the seed, roots, and whole plant to treat coughs, flatulence, jaundice, colic, gout, joint pain, parasites, and general inflammation.

Cannabis and the New World

By the time the New World was being colonized, cannabis had become an integral part of the European economy. With the explosion of maritime trade, hemp's mass production began in Italy's powerful port of Venice where it was made into some of the world's finest ropes and sails. Other European maritime powers like Portugal, Spain, England, and the Netherlands had huge demands for hemp, as well.

Explorers and colonizers arrived on the shores of the New World on sails made of hemp. It is believed that conquistador Pedro Cuadrado, in service to Hernando Cortés, was the first European to bring hemp seeds to the Western Hemisphere for cultivation. The Spanish colony of Chile started cultivating cannabis in 1545 in an effort to reduce their dependence on Russian hemp, Russia developing a near monopoly on hemp production at that time.

Cannabis was introduced to North America via Nova Scotia in 1606 by the French botanist and apothecary Louis Hebert, who became Canada's first apothecary. In 1607, the first British colony was established in Jamestown, Virginia, and was required to grow hemp to help their government back home reduce their reliance on Russian hemp. By 1611, King James had made cultivation mandatory, despite the fact that colonists preferred to grow food and tobacco, which fetched higher prices. In 1619, it was demanded that every colony household grow 100 plants, and by 1630 most colonist clothing was made from hemp. In 1632, Connecticut made growing hemp mandatory, followed shortly by Massachusetts. In 1682, farmers were allowed to pay off debt with hemp, and in 1735, Massachusetts residents were allowed to pay their taxes in hemp.

By the time the Revolutionary War began in 1775, the American colonies had become proficient in spinning and textile making, and no longer relied on their colonial powers to sell these products (made from their own hemp) back to them. They began selling their products to France, a major trade rival and military rival of Britain. They used the money from these exports for weaponry. It is believed that Thomas Jefferson's first drafts of the Declaration of Independence were written on hemp paper.

Hemp crops were instrumental in helping our forefathers succeed in colonizing America. With the ability to make clothes, towels, paper, and other products, the original settlers were not only encouraged, but at key points in our history required, to cultivate hemp. Hemp production helped America sever ties with Great Britain; hemp became integral to the colonists' way of life.

Forefathers and their Hemp Fields

There have been tall tales about George Washington, James Madison, and James Monroe smoking cannabis and hashish. While there is no solid historical record for these claims, we do know that both Washington and Jefferson grew hemp along with many of their fellow Americans. Washington grew hemp on all five of his farms at Mount Vernon, Virginia, as did Jefferson at his Monticello plantation.

Even after America had gained independence, cannabis continued to be an important part of the economy. While the monetary system went through its initial development, counterfeiting was a major problem. Hemp, with its reliable quality and continued demand, was used as currency to bridge the gap. But by the early 19th century, cultivation of cannabis in America slowed. Not only was production of hemp difficult and time-consuming, but by then cotton was fetching much higher prices and wood was being used more and more in paper production. And the very sails that cannabis had rode in on were being replaced by steamships.

The Victorian Age Medical Revival

As a medicine, hemp was a familiar ingredient in Asian and Indian folk remedies; something of a cure-all, used for fever, burns, and headaches, as well as a paste/poultice for wounds. By way of an Irish doctor working in India, hashish made it back to Europe as a medicine.

While working for The East India Company in Bengal, William Brooke O'Shaughnessy observed the local use of hashish and began to experiment to see if it had therapeutic properties. Initially he fed it to dogs, and then humans. He found it worked very well as a sedative and anticonvulsant, and wrote several papers detailing his research. O'Shaughnessy is credited with introducing cannabis to Western medicine.

In 1842, he gave some hashish to the British pharmacist Peter Squire, who used high-proof alcohol to make a tincture. He patented the tincture as an analgesic (pain reliever) called Squire's Extract, which was sold throughout Europe and the

Americas. Doctors were eager to have a painkiller to replace opium, and Squire's extract quickly caught on across England, where pharmacists began making their own preparations. Well-known companies like Eli Lilly, Parke-Davis, and Bayer produced tinctures that contained cannabis, which were considered safe and effective for conditions of nausea, delirium, epilepsy, migraine, and painful spasms.

Through the late 1800s, cannabis extracts found their way onto apothecary shelves and into doctors' bags. According to Dr. Ethan Russo, Director of Research and Development at the International Cannabis and Cannabinoids Institute, historically cannabis was used for therapeutic purposes primarily in the form of teas, extracts, and tinctures (grains of hemp/hashish resin dissolved in alcohol)—not in smoked form; and that during this time, the composition of the resin would have been about equal parts THC and CBD.

From 1851 through 1941, Extractum Cannabis (cannabis extract) was listed in the *US Pharmacopeià*. With each edition, the definition of cannabis was expanded as well as the uses it had medicinally. For those unfamiliar with this tome, the *US Pharmacopeia* was first published in 1920, its purpose to identify and standardize the drugs that are in medical use. In its earliest editions the majority of its listings were botanical in nature, as many of our pharmaceuticals today have a history in plants and herbs. Today the *Pharmacopeia* stands as a written physical reference for standards in medicines, food ingredients, dietary supplement products, and ingredients.

As these tinctures made their way across the Atlantic and into American pharmacies, doctors used them to treat everything from tonsillitis to tetanus to snake bites. Dr. E. A. Birch formally recommended its use for treating opium withdrawal in the esteemed medical journal *The Lancet*. Tinctures were available without a prescription, were inexpensive, and came to be considered to something of a "cure-all." But the potency of these medicinal preparations was variable and individual responses unpredictable and erratic; the inconsistency of the medicines was attributed to the limited technology of that time period along with the considerable variability of the plants.

Because of this variability in strength, cannabis tinctures were soon replaced by the newest drug to hit pharmacy shelves: aspirin. Predictable and consistent, aspirin promised to be the painkiller of the future.

CANNABIS DOCTOR TO THE QUEEN

Sir John Russell Reynolds was a famous doctor in Victorian Era England. He had a very prestigious career, the highlight of which was perhaps serving as doctor to Queen Victoria. In 1890, he published a paper called "On the Therapeutic Uses and Toxic Effects of *Cannabis indica*." He was aware of the unpredictable strength of various tinctures and recommended that people begin with small doses to gauge the strength. It is rumored he prescribed Queen Victoria cannabis tincture as a painkiller for menstrual cramps. While there is no direct account of this happening, it's not entirely impossible that it did. At the time there was no stigma attached to using cannabis medicinally.

Cannabis in the Post-Prohibition Era

Although cannabis has a rich history as a medicine in many countries around the world, including the United States, the political climate of the early 20th century was not cannabis or hemp friendly, providing a perfect storm for cannabis prohibition, with the mingling of unstable medicine, racism, greed, and power.

By the end of the 19th century, cannabis cultivation and use was on the decline in the Western world. Steamships were replacing hemp-made sails, and doctors were favoring the consistency of chemically synthesized pharmaceuticals like aspirin. When the Pure Food and Drug Act was passed in 1906, stricter labeling requirements meant people began seeing cannabis listed alongside opium and cocaine in many tinctures. With widespread opium addiction already a concern, cannabis began to be associated with narcotics.

When the Mexican Revolution began in 1910, Mexicans fleeing the war brought with them rolled cannabis leaves and flowers, which they called marijuana. Soon businesses in Texas and New Mexico were importing cannabis, and it was available in grocery stores. It was used primarily among workers to unwind and relax, allowing them to wake up in the morning without the hangover associated with alcohol. Its popularity and recreational use spread.

Fast forward to the 1930s when the prohibition of alcohol ended. The Federal Bureau of Narcotics (FBN) was founded, and Harry J. Anslinger was appointed as director. Anslinger had an impressive track record of thwarting alcohol and drug smugglers overseas. With a full department and time on his hands due to Prohibition ending, Anslinger needed a target to keep the FBN staff working and maintain a line item in the government's yearly budget. Anslinger decided his mission would be to rid the US of all drugs, including cannabis.

WHAT WAS PROHIBITION?

According to History.com, the ratification of the 18th Amendment to the US Constitution—which banned the manufacture, transportation, and sale of intoxicating liquors—ushered in a period in American history known as Prohibition. The temperance movement was widespread during the first decade of the 20th century, with temperance societies a common fixture in communities across the United States. Women played a strong role in the temperance movement, as alcohol was seen as a destructive force in families and marriages, with saloon culture viewed as corrupt and ungodly. Many factory owners also supported Prohibition, looking to prevent on-the-job accidents and increase the efficiency of their workers in an era of increased industrial production and extended working hours.

Reefer Madness

Anslinger took advantage of the skeptical and racist rumblings around cannabis that had been surfacing in the media during the 1930s and launched his own targeted campaign against marijuana with the aim of making it illegal. He associated marijuana with poor minority populations, immoral behavior, and monstrous acts. Anslinger found support from the nationwide Hearst newspaper chain, which frequently ran stories of "insanity, criminality, and death" caused by smoking marijuana. He circulated pamphlets and articles about the dangers of smoking cannabis, and published the famous article titled "Marihuana: Assassin of Youth," which warned parents about the perils of marijuana.

Films like *Reefer Madness* (1936), *Marihuana: Assassin of Youth* (1935), and *Marihuana: The Devil's Weed* (1936) were propaganda designed to gain public support so that anti-marijuana laws could be passed. A tide of hysteria swept the nation.

In 1937, Congress enacted the Marihuana Tax Act, which effectively made it impossible to possess cannabis for recreational use. The American Medical Association testified that cannabis was not the dangerous narcotic that Anslinger and the media was making it out to be, but since Dr. William Woodward was really the only voice from the AMA to defend the findings, the bill passed easily.

The Marihuana Tax Act of 1937 regulated the importation, cultivation, possession, and/or distribution of marijuana. The Act made the possession and sale of cannabis a lengthy and bureaucratically difficult endeavor, requiring registration fees, various documents, and stamps of approval. Violation of the act resulted in a fine of up to $2,000 and/or imprisonment for up to five years.

In principle, the Marihuana Tax Act of 1937 stopped only the use of the plant as a recreational drug. In practice, though, industrial hemp was caught up in the anti-marijuana legislation, making hemp importation and commercial production in this country less economical. Scientific research and medical testing of marijuana also virtually disappeared at this time.

The Jazz Era Dealer Was White

As jazz grew in popularity, it spread north from its home in New Orleans, and cannabis went with it. Though the negative stereotype of the weed-smoking jazz musician was generally that of a black man, it was actually a white jazz musician that spread cannabis in the jazz scene.

Milton "Mezz" Mezzrow first came across cannabis in a club in Indiana in 1924, and he brought it with him when he moved to Harlem in the 1930s. There, he became well-known for selling cannabis to many of the most famous jazz musicians (all of which Harry Anslinger was keeping tabs on); Louis Armstrong is reported to be one of his biggest customers. Armstrong (among several other prominent jazz artists) even penned a song about cannabis called "Muggles," a slang term for cannabis at the time.

He became so well-known for selling cannabis that Mezz actually became slang for cannabis among jazz musicians, and it was widely available in jazz clubs. Cannabis was also available in "tea pads," or apartments in New York where people would gather to consume cannabis together. After the Marihuana Tax Act was passed, Mezzrow was arrested and ended his career as a dealer.

Mayor of New York Supports Cannabis

When Anslinger began coming down hard on cannabis with the Marihuana Tax Act, the mayor of New York City at the time, Fiorello La Guardia, decided to investigate further. He was both concerned about reports of cannabis spreading in his city and skeptical that it was as bad as Anslinger was making it out to be.

He commissioned the New York Academy of Medicine to investigate. In 1944, after five years of studying the psychological, physical, and sociological effects of cannabis use, they published "The Marihuana Problem in the City of New York" and concluded that cannabis had no addictive qualities, nor did it lead to addiction to other narcotics. It also concluded that use of cannabis was not a problem among the youth of New York City and had little to do with crime. Anslinger dismissed the report as "medical mumbo-jumbo." He threatened to arrest anyone who used cannabis in their research.

The Beats and the Hippies

The 1950s saw the Beat subculture spring up around writers and artists like Jack Kerouac, Alan Ginsberg, and William S. Burroughs. They became infamous for their drug use, which included cannabis. The Beats were embraced by young rebels who questioned the established norms of society.

At the same time, public opinion on cannabis had softened, and it was no longer viewed as absolutely harmful. Despite the findings of the La Guardia report that cannabis did not lead to the use of narcotics, Anslinger totally pursued that angle while taking advantage of public fears around the increasing use of heroin and cocaine.

In 1951, The Boggs Act was passed into law, which mandated minimum sentencing for drug possession. The Narcotics Control Act of 1956 would mandate even harsher penalties.

And still, cultural support for cannabis rolled on. While cannabis might be a tried-and-true hippie stereotype, during the '60s there were countless flower-clad college kids smoking joints across the country. Their galvanizing force was protesting the Vietnam War and cannabis helped them spread feelings of "peace and love, man." At the same time, soldiers returning from war sought out cannabis, as it was widely available overseas.

Cannabis continued to be found throughout music and art, with figures like John Lennon, Eric Clapton, Bob Dylan, Bob Marley, and David Bowie picking up arrests for it, and iconic events like Woodstock serving as an artistic and cultural distillation of the movement.

The War on Drugs

The "War on Drugs" was a term popularized by the media during Richard Nixon's presidency, when in 1971 he declared drug abuse "public enemy number one." On October 27, 1970, Nixon signed the Controlled Substances Act (CSA) into law. What this did was put the federal government in charge of "overseeing the manufacture, importation, possession, use, and distribution of certain narcotics, stimulants, depressants, hallucinogens, anabolic steroids, and other chemicals."

Even today, Food and Drug Administration (FDA) employees with backgrounds in medicine and science follow guidelines developed in 1970 to determine how safe pharmaceutical medicines are and how easy it is for healthcare practitioners to prescribe or recommend them. The CSA can and has been amended over the years, but the processes and guidelines have remained consistent. It classifies drugs into five categories depending on their safety, their use, and their abuse potential. For example, over-the-counter medicines vs. something you need to get filled by your pharmacist.

According to the United States Drug Enforcement Administration's website, the abuse rate is a determinate factor in the scheduling of drugs. "Schedule I drugs have a high potential for abuse and the potential to create severe psychological and/or physical dependence. As the drug schedule changes—Schedule II, Schedule III, etc., so does the abuse potential—Schedule V drugs represent the least potential for abuse."

Unlike prohibition of alcohol, which restricted the manufacturing and distribution—not the possession—marijuana laws have consistently outlawed the production, sale, possession, and consumption of the drug. Today, the Controlled Substances Act of 1970 designates cannabis as a Schedule I drug by the Drug Enforcement Administration (DEA), meaning:

(A) The drug or other substance has a high potential for abuse.

(B) The drug or other substance has no currently accepted medical use in treatment in the United States.

(C) There is a lack of accepted safety for use of the drug or other substance under medical supervision.

So as a Schedule I drug, cannabis is considered to have no medical value and has a high potential for abuse, along with other drugs like LSD, ecstasy, and peyote. This classification continues as of this writing to produce a labyrinth of legal and institutional obstacles that prohibit research, prevent the therapeutic use of cannabis medicines, and keep both drug and fiber types of cannabis prohibited under federal law, as the distinction between hemp and cannabis continue to be largely unrecognized.

In 1975, the National Commission on Marihuana and Drug Abuse (also known as the Shafer Commission) published the "White Paper on Drug Abuse: A Report to the President." The report concluded cannabis was a "low-priority drug," that it was not addictive, and it did not lead to the consumption of harder narcotics. It recommended that cannabis be considered the least priority of drug enforcement officials. This information went ignored by then President Nixon.

First Lady Nancy Reagan became the face for the antidrug sentiment with the popular Just Say No campaign that kicked off in 1982. By 1986 the Antidrug Abuse Act had been passed, which reinstated minimum drug sentences and contained the infamous three-strikes policy that led to life imprisonment without parole after three felony drug offenses.

Incarceration rates exploded. To this day minorities, particularly black minorities, are disproportionately jailed for drug offenses even though cannabis use among black and white people is roughly even (14 and 12 percent, respectively). Black people are 3.7 times more likely to be arrested for possession according to the American Civil Liberties Union (ACLU).

Decade of the Brain and Medical Legalization

By the late '80s and early '90s, research on the medical uses of cannabis was still fairly limited, both here and abroad. Research efforts at the time were largely directed by the National Institute on Drug Abuse (NIDA), which was subsidizing studies to uncover the damaging effects of THC and cannabis. Medical-grade cannabis for research purposes was (and continues to be) available only through one single grow house at the University of Mississippi.

Little did NIDA know, their research would lead to some of the most exciting discoveries we've made about the human brain—discoveries that would explode into what became known as "the Decade of the Brain" among brain researchers and scientists.

During the 1990s, there were more advances in neuroscience than in all previous years combined! Not only did our understanding of the brain advance by leaps and bounds, but we also came to understand the underlying mechanisms for many different forms of disease. All thanks to cannabis.

But let's dial it back for a second. In 1964, Dr. Raphael Mechoulam, along with colleague Yehiel Gaoni, first identified and then synthesized tetrahyrdocannabinol (THC). This was a *major* step forward in cannabis medicine, and Mechoulam is widely recognized as the "grandfather of cannabis science." For decades after this, nearly all cannabis research

HEALING WITH CBD

revolved around THC. During this time, we developed a fairly good understanding of what THC was—its pharmacology, biochemistry, and clinical effects—but we didn't understand how it worked in the brain at the molecular level to stimulate appetite, relieve pain, or alter consciousness.

In a government-funded study done through the St. Louis University School of Medicine in 1988, scientists Allyn Howlett and William Devane first identified that the brain had specialized receptors for cannabinoids, and it turned out that the brain contained more of these receptors than any other. Using a potent form of synthetic THC, researchers were able to map where these receptors were, and discovered they were most concentrated in the areas responsible for mental and physical processes: the hippocampus (memory), cerebral cortex (higher cognition), cerebellum (motor coordination), basal ganglia (movement), hypothalamus (appetite), and amygdala (emotions).

Then in 1990, Lisa Matsuda and her colleagues at the National Institute of Mental Health (NIMH) announced they had cloned the THC receptor (called the CB1 receptor). This was crucial, because it meant that researchers could begin sculpting "keys" to turn the receptors' "locks." In 1993, a second cannabinoid receptor, called the CB2 receptor, was discovered and cloned. This receptor is found primarily in the immune system and peripheral nervous system. CB2 receptors are also present in the gut, spleen, liver, heart, kidneys, bones, blood vessels, lymph cells, endocrine glands, and reproductive organs.

The next major discovery in cannabis would come from Mechoulam, in collaboration with the NIMH, who discovered that our bodies produce their own cannabis-like compound that binds to the same CB1 receptors as THC: N-arachidonoylethanolamine or AEA, more commonly known as anandamide, and named after the Sanskrit word for "bliss." Soon after, Mechoulam and his colleagues would discover a second endocannabinoid, 2-arachidonoylglycerol or 2-AG, which interacts with both the CB1 and CB2 receptors.

The discovery of receptors that are uniquely designed to interact with chemical compounds in cannabis, added to the discovery that our own bodies produce compounds similar to THC, ushered humanity into another MAJOR discovery: the endocannabinoid system, named after the plant that led to its discovery. This system is likely to have started developing in life on Earth 600 million years ago, and is present in fish, reptiles, earthworms, amphibians, birds, and mammals, and serves a very crucial and basic function in animal physiology: maintaining homeostasis. (See Chapter 3: The Endocannabinoid System for more).

According to Martin Lee, author and founder of Project CBD, "advances in the burgeoning field of cannabinoid studies would pave the way for new treatment strategies for various pathological conditions—cancer, diabetes, neuropathic pain, arthritis, osteoporosis, obesity, Alzheimer's, multiple sclerosis, depression, and many other diseases that seemed beyond the reach of conventional cures."

Other experiments would establish that cannabinoid receptors (CB1, CB2) modulate pain, inflammation, appetite, gastrointestinal motility, and sleep cycles, along with the ebb and flow of immune cells, hormones, and other mood-altering neurotransmitters such as **serotonin**, **dopamine**, and **glutamate**.

What Are Cannabinoids?

Cannabinoids are active and medicinally beneficial compounds in both cannabis and hemp plants. They help our bodies maintain balance (homeostasis) and are similar in function to endogenous cannabinoids, which the body makes itself (see Chapter 3: The Endocannabinoid System). The most well-known cannabinoid is THC, while CBD has recently ignited the interest of both the public and scientific communities for its non-impairing therapeutic benefits. But there are over 100 other cannabinoids, most of which we know very little about. Several of these cannabinoids and their acidic varieties will be discussed in this book. See also Chapter 4: Cannabinoids and The Entourage Effect for more.

Among growing incarceration rates and the exciting new research into the medical uses of cannabis, people began to question the wisdom of cannabis laws. The tide of public support for medicinal use swelled. In 1996, California passed Proposition 215, also known as the Compassionate Use Act, to allow for medical use. In 1998, Alaska, Oregon, and Washington followed suit, and today (as of this writing), 30 states have medical programs.

There is an interesting level of inconsistency in the federal government's stance on cannabis. As a Schedule I drug, cannabis has "no currently accepted medical use in treatment in the United States." And yet, the federal government's National Institutes of Health (NIH) holds a patent for medical use. Issued in 2003, Patent #6,630,507 (often referred to Patent '507) covers the key medicinal properties of cannabis and calls out CBD specifically as being a potent antioxidant and neuroprotectant, along with being very safe for human consumption.

The abstract states:

"The cannabinoids are found to have particular application as neuroprotectants, for example in limiting neurological damage following ischemic [deficient supply of blood] insults, such as stroke and trauma, or in the treatment of neurodegenerative diseases, such as Alzheimer's disease, Parkinson's disease, and HIV dementia. Non-psychoactive cannabinoids, such as cannabidiol, are particularly advantageous to use because they avoid toxicity that is encountered with psychoactive cannabinoids at high doses."

Patent '507 protects the use of cannabinoids "as antioxidant compounds and compositions...that act as free radical scavengers" and "in the prevention and treatment of pathological conditions...due to cardiovascular and neurovascular conditions and neurodegenerative diseases." The patent incorporates "free radical associated disease" such as:

- ischemia (tissue hypoxia), ischemia/reperfusion injury, and myocardial ischemia or infarction

- inflammatory diseases and systemic lupus erythematosus

- cerebrovascular accidents (like stroke) and spinal cord trauma

- Down's syndrome

- Crohn's disease

- autoimmune diseases (like rheumatoid arthritis or diabetes)

- cataract formation and uveitis

- emphysema

- gastric ulcers

- oxygen toxicity

- neoplasia or undesired cellular apoptosis

- radiation sickness

According to the patent, central nervous system diseases, particularly Parkinson's disease, Alzheimer's disease, HIV dementia, and autoimmune neurodegenerative disease such as encephalitis and hypoxia may experience a benefit from the antioxidative properties exerted by cannabinoids.

That's quite a comprehensive list for a drug that has no acknowledged medical value! It's clear that denying the medical value of cannabis is more of a political act than a scientific determination.

The current catch-22 of cannabis science here in the US is that because it is a Schedule I drug it can't easily be studied. But because it hasn't been thoroughly investigated, it remains a Schedule I drug. Despite the situation here, much research is being done abroad, with countries like Israel (helmed by Dr. Mechoulam) leading the charge. Israel has become the epicenter of cannabis research, and many American companies outsource research to labs in Israel because it's so difficult to do adequate research here. Other countries like China and Iran are also doing extensive work on studying the endocannabinoid system.

Adult-Use Legalization

As medicinal use becomes more and more commonplace and approval for medical cannabis has become nearly unanimous, the public increasingly sees cannabis as safe to consume. In 2012, the first adult-use (also called "recreational use") laws were passed by ballot in Colorado and Washington.

As of this writing, 9 states plus the District of Columbia have legalized cannabis for recreational or adult-use:

1. Alaska
2. California
3. Colorado
4. District of Columbia
5. Maine
6. Massachusetts
7. Nevada
8. Oregon
9. Vermont
10. Washington

While most adult-use states are fairly new and working out the kinks around licensing, setting up dispensaries, distribution, and banking, the money has begun to pour in: Sales hit $9 billion in 2017 and the industry employed over 120,000 people.

Recent Research: 2016 Onward

As of this writing, there are over 140 active clinical studies looking at the medicinal application of cannabidiol. Just head on over to ClinicalTrials.gov for a current listing of studies that are in process. A search of PubMed.gov, a database of scientific studies and reviews maintained by the US National Library of Medicine, National Institutes of Health, will yield over 500 such papers in the last two years alone. In the world of CBD research, things are moving and shaking!

Research from 2016 onward has focused heavily on taking a deeper dive into neurodegenerative diseases like ALS, Parkinson's, Huntington's, Alzheimer's, and MS. Several studies have looked at CBD's role in mitigating the symptoms of, and even reversing, dementia. Dementia is one of the most debilitating and hard-to-manage symptoms across several neurodegenerative diseases. The neuroprotectant qualities of CBD are being looked at not just in the context of neurodegenerative diseases, but also as possible prevention and treatment of stroke.

The broader uses of CBD to treat addiction are becoming clear, too, with research looking at CBD's effects on opioid use and withdrawal, alcoholism, cannabis use disorder, and cocaine addiction. Some study has also looked at CBD's effect on reducing craving and withdrawal symptoms in general.

The same is true of psychiatric disorders, a wide umbrella that includes schizophrenia, bipolar disorder, generalized anxiety disorder, and depression. Several studies have looked at CBD as an antipsychotic medicine, which would make it useful for schizophrenia and bipolar disorder. CBD is also being looked at as an effective way of combating anhedonia, which would help patients suffering from depression find happiness in activities they once enjoyed doing.

There continues to be a huge push in looking at CBD and seizure disorders, with lots of preclinical work still being done and research moving into more and more human clinical trials. PTSD and fear-based memory are areas of interest at the preclinical level, as are diabetes, inflammatory bowel conditions, neuropathic pain, and nausea.

Are All Research Studies Created Equally?

The current system to take a drug from research and development to human consumption goes something like this: New drugs go through various stages of study before being approved for public consumption. Each round of study offers more and more credibility in terms of the promise of the drug's efficacy in human patients. After initial discovery work to identify a compound and therapeutic target for the compound, studies are carried out in laboratories and typically involve looking at the effects of a drug on cells of tissue or flesh in a test tube (in vitro). This initial step in the development process is considered least credible in terms of ultimate usability. Next, live animal subjects will be tested (in vivo). While results from these studies can be promising, often the results aren't the same for human subjects. These two initial testing phases are called "preclinical trials." From here, the next tier up in terms of credibility are reviews. For reviews, researchers will compile all relevant studies on a particular condition, evaluate each study, and draw conclusions based on this broader base of data. Reviews are more credible than any individual laboratory or animal study, but are middle-of-the-road in terms of credibility. Not surprisingly, the most credible support for a drug comes from human trials, also called "clinical trials." There are a variety of ways clinical trials can be designed and carried out. Controlled human clinical trials offer fairly solid evidence, and randomized double-blind placebo-controlled studies are considered the most credible as far as efficacy and success rates are concerned. In a randomized double-blind, placebo-controlled trial, some of the participants are given the treatment being studied while others are given a fake treatment (a placebo). Neither the researchers nor the participants know which is which until the study ends (they are thus both "blind").

Current Clinical Trials

Human clinical trials are where we get to really understand the efficacy of CBD. As of this writing there are clinical trials looking at CBD specifically for:

- Alcohol use disorder (alcoholism)

- Bipolar disorder

- Cervical cancer

- Cocaine addiction

- Epilepsy

- Graft-versus-host disease

- Infantile spasms (a form of seizure disorder)

- Multiple sclerosis

- Prader-Willi syndrome (a genetic disorder affecting appetite, growth, metabolism, cognitive function, and behavior)

- Schizophrenia

- Sturge-Weber syndrome (a neurological disorder)

And there are many others! There are also clinical trials looking at CBD's ability to counteract the effects of long-term

THC use, like memory loss and depression. Research is also looking at the effects of early adoption of heavy cannabis use on adolescent brains, and how CBD might help mitigate damaging effects. There is a flip side to every coin, and while it's important to look at the positive effects CBD might have on the human body and disease, it's also important to understand how cannabis might negatively impact us as well.

New and Exciting Areas of Research

On the horizon, there are exciting new preclinical studies looking at how CBD might treat conditions like endometrial and cervical cancer (there are lots of cannabinoid receptors in the female reproductive system!), panic attacks, and a pediatric form of cancer called neuroblastoma. Italian researchers are also proposing an expanded understanding of the endocannabinoid system that they are calling the "endocannabinoidome," which includes the family of endogenous cannabinoids and other active compounds that act like endogenous cannabinoids, along with all receptors they interact with (not just CB1 and CB2) and the enzymes that create and break the compounds down.[1]

CHAPTER 3

The Endocannabinoid System

"By using a plant that has been around for thousands of years, we discovered a new physiological system of immense importance. We wouldn't have been able to get there if we had not looked at the plant."

—Dr. Raphael Mechoulam

So let's just get this out there from the start: Human beings (actually, more accurately, fish, reptiles, earthworms, leeches, amphibians, birds, and all mammals including human beings), have a built-in, biological system that can receive, process, and use the medicinal compounds in cannabis. In other words, we are hardwired to use these compounds.

You might be thinking, "Say whaaaaaat?" Yes! It's true! But it's not something most people (or most doctors for that matter) even know about, despite the fact that it is legitimately one of the most important discoveries science has made about how the human body functions and mitigates disease. Now you might be thinking, "Huh? How does that even make sense?" Sadly, it makes sense if you understand the social history of cannabis, which is a very complicated tale worth familiarizing yourself with. It was covered in Chapter 2: A Brief History of Cannabis, but if you jumped ahead, be sure to check it out—we promise it won't disappoint!

But let's get back to the fascinating discovery of this system that resides right inside you at this very moment. Hopefully the chapter title was a tip-off, it's called the endogenous cannabinoid system (or endocannabinoid system), an innate bodily system that produces its own cannabinoid-like compounds and can process the cannabinoids found in hemp and cannabis. According to Dr. John McPartland this system started developing in life on Earth around 600 million years ago.

While we started looking at cannabis from a medicinal lens thousands of years ago, things didn't really get cooking until about 125 years ago when we started isolating individual **cannabinoids** in cannabis. **Cannabinol** (CBN, see page 72 for more) came first in 1895, followed by cannabidiol (CBD) in 1940 and the mother lode of cannabinoid discoveries, **tetrahyrdocannabinol**, or THC, in 1964, by revered cannabis researcher and pharmacologist Dr. Raphael Mechoulam.

The Big Picture

"The discovery of the endocannabinoid system (ECS) is the single most important scientific medical discovery since the recognition of sterile surgical technique. As our knowledge expands, we are coming to realize

that the ECS is a master control system of virtually all physiology."

—Dr. David B. Allen

The endogenous cannabinoid system is an extensive network of neurons, neural pathways, receptors, cells, molecules, and enzymes that work tirelessly throughout your body to maintain a state of **homeostasis**: a stable internal environment despite fluctuations in the external environment.

The ECS is essential to life's basic processes by relaying messages that affect how we "relax, eat, sleep, forget, and protect," as noted by the Italian researcher Vincenzo Di Marzo, Research Director at the Institute of Biomolecular Chemistry of the National Research Council and editor of several books on cannabinoids.

So in other words, it's responsible for two major functions in the body: modulating pleasure, energy, and well-being while restoring bodily balance in the face of external stressors (physical, emotional, and psychological). The total effect of the ECS is to regulate homeostasis and prevent disease and aging.

Seems like a pretty important system, no? And yet, a 2013 survey of 157 accredited American medical schools (carried out by Dr. David B. Allen, a retired cardiothoracic and vascular surgeon and endocannabinoid researcher), showed that only 13% of medical schools mentioned the endocannabinoid system in curriculum. Today's physicians weren't taught that cannabis can be a medicine; they were taught that it was a drug of abuse.

So how does the ECS fit into the big the picture of our body's complex inner workings? And why is it important to the mitigation of disease?

Let's explain by looking at one specific bodily system, the immune system. Say your body is faced with a virus or bacterial invader. Your immune system will kick on like a furnace to produce the fever needed to fry the invader. When the job is done, the ECS signals the immune system to cool down and restore homeostasis. But if the feedback loop is out of control, if the immune system overreacts to stress or mistakes its own body for a foreign invader, this is when we develop autoimmune diseases or inflammatory disorders.

According to Dr. Robert Melamede, a biologist that devoted his career to the study of the endocannabinoid system, you can think of the ECS as the task master that is constantly multitasking, adjusting, and readjusting the complex network of molecular thermostats that control our physiological tempo—and you'll remember that our bodies like to keep this tempo balanced.

The ECS is unique because of its "retrograde signaling," which is how it helps bodies maintain homeostasis. **Retrograde signaling** is what's happening when the ECS tells your immune system to cool it after a fever has done its work, for example. According to Martin Lee, it is a form of intracellular communication that inhibits immune response, reduces inflammation, relaxes muscles, lowers blood pressure, dilates bronchial passages, and normalizes overstimulated nerves. And as Lee explains, "retrograde signaling serves as an inhibitory feedback mechanism that tells other neurotransmitters to cool it when they are firing too fast."

And let's not forget how we came to understand these inner workings in the first place: cannabis! The cannabinoids in hemp and cannabis stimulate the same receptors (CB1 and CB2) that our own natural compounds do, serving as a substitute "retrograde messenger" that mimics just what our bodies do when they try to maintain balance. This gives cannabis a unique synergy with our own bodily processes, and allows it to be a natural and nontoxic medicine. It is also why cannabis-based treatments and supplements must be tailored to the individual, because everybody and every ECS is unique.

Not only that, but the endocannabinoid system is not a lone wolf, meaning it is not a self-contained system. The ECS interacts robustly with other non-cannabinoid systems like the endorphin system, the immune system, and the vanilloid system (responsible for changing pain from acute to chronic). In modulating these other systems, the ECS regulates inflammation, pain, bone health, formation of new nerve cells, fat and sugar processing, mood, energy, brain health, and hormone balance.

Next, let's talk about the most important parts of the endocannabinoid system in a little more detail.

Endogenous Cannabinoids and Phytocannabinoids

The chemical messengers we talked about earlier, the ones that the ECS sends to cool your system down in the fever example, are what we call **neurotransmitters**. Cannabinoids, both the ones our body produces itself and the ones we get from cannabis, are neurotransmitters. There are hundreds of different neurotransmitters produced by the body for use in the specific systems they're needed.

Endogenous cannabinoids (or endocannabinoids) are compounds that our body produces itself. Your body creates endocannabinoids with the help of fatty acids. Omega-3 fatty acids are especially important for this, and research in animals has shown a connection between diets low in omega-3s and mood changes caused by poor endocannabinoid regulation. Hemp seeds are a quality source of omega-3, but fish like salmon and sardines produce a form of omega-3s that is easier for your body to use. Nuts and eggs are also good sources of omega-3s. New research has found that omega-3s fatty acids might also provide anti-inflammatory benefits in much the same way as our endocannabinoids and the cannabinoids in hemp and cannabis do.[2]

The two endocannabinoids we know of were discovered by Dr. Raphael Mechoulam and his colleagues. They are produced "on demand" by nerve cells (called neurons) whenever our ECS needs to kick on to maintain balance. They tell your body when to get certain processes started, and when to stop them. The first endocannabinoid, N-arachidonoylethanolamine (AEA), is more commonly known as anandamide. The second is 2-arachidonoylglycerol, or 2-AG.

When picked up by the specialized cannabinoid receptors that sit on our cells, endocannabinoids give the cell specific directions. It might be to reduce inflammation in your gut or mitigate the pain response when you stub your toe. Regardless of the reason the ECS kicks on, the goal is to help the body get back to a state of homeostasis, and the production of endocannabinoids helps regulate this process. We now understand that by controlling the volume at which neurotransmitters are sent, cannabinoids can impact the length and intensity of the body's response.

Your ECS, Diet, and Lifestyle

A great way to approach supporting your ECS in general is through diet.[3] A diet that emphasizes greens, beans, onions, mushrooms, berries, and seeds (or a G-BOMB diet) is not only good for your ECS but your body as a whole because these foods are the most nutrient-dense and health-promoting foods on the planet.

Another way to support your ECS is through lifestyle: massage, acupuncture, exercise, and weight control can all upregulate (or enhance) your endocannabinoid system.[4] The effects of stress can deplete the ECS as well, and so active stress management through yoga, meditation, and deep breathing can be beneficial in maintaining a vital system.[5] Moderate- to high-intensity exercise also increases endocannabinoid levels (particularly anandamide) in the body, supporting previous research that has shown exercise has anti-depressant–like effects.[6]

As mentioned, phytocannabinoids are cannabinoids that come from plants. These plant cannabinoids (like THC, CBD) stimulate our cannabinoid receptors and carry out functions similar to our own endogenous anandamide and 2-AG.

THC is the most thoroughly understood phytocannabinoid because its psychoactive effects garnered it the attention it needed to be studied extensively. CBD is a relative newcomer on the "hot topics of cannabis science" list, so we know less about it. There are over 100 other phytocannabinoids present in cannabis just waiting to be understood and studied for their medicinal potential. Phytocannabinoids bind to both the CB1 and CB2 receptors and interact with them in similar ways as anandamide and 2-AG do.

Cannabinoids Are a Natural Defense for Cannabis

Interestingly, the cannabis plant also uses THC and other cannabinoids to promote its own health and prevent disease. Cannabinoids have antioxidant properties that protect the leaves and flowering structures from ultraviolet radiation; they neutralize the harmful free radicals generated by UV rays, protecting the cells. In humans, free radicals cause aging, cancer, and impaired healing. Antioxidants found in plants have long been promoted as natural supplements to prevent free radical harm.

We also know that non-psychoactive phytocannabinoids from other plants, and even other **phytochemicals**, or active plant compounds like terpenes and flavonoids, can be picked up and utilized by receptors in our endocannabinoid systems.

But unlike our endocannabinoids, there are no enzymes present in the body that can immediately break down phytocannabinoids and, therefore, their effects last much longer. When consuming cannabis-based medicines, the body gets much higher levels of cannabinoids than it can produce itself, thus producing a therapeutic effect. In addition to this, CBD blocks the enzyme that breaks down AEA and THC, which in effect increases our "endocannabinoid tone."

As described by neurologist and subject expert Dr. Ethan Russo, there is "a hypothesis that all humans have an underlying endocannabinoid tone that is a reflection of the levels of anandamide and 2-AG, their production, metabolism, and the relative abundance and state of cannabinoid receptors." A compromised endocannabinoid tone may result in illness and disease, including clinical endocannabinoid deficiency.

Clinical endocannabinoid deficiency (or CECD) was first proposed by Dr. Ethan Russo in 2004 and more recently investigated by Steele Clark Smith and Mark S. Wagner in 2014. The main idea is simple: When the body does not produce enough endocannabinoids or cannot regulate them properly, you are more susceptible to illnesses that affect one or several of the functions overseen by the endocannabinoid system (see Receptors and Physiology of the ECS). Endocannabinoid deficiencies could be the root cause of many autoimmune disorders like migraines, fibromyalgia, and irritable bowel syndrome (IBS). One possible solution might be microdosing. Because small doses of phytocannabinoids can encourage the body to create more naturally occurring endocannabinoids and their receptors, it may be possible to boost our systems and avoid deficiencies with regular small doses of phytocannabinoids like CBD, THC, and CBN. Small doses tend to perturb our CB1 and CB2 receptors with the effect of boosting production of our own natural endocannabinoids.

Synthetic Cannabinoids

Synthetic versions of both THC and CBD have been developed. THC has been modified to create synthetic analog drugs like HU-210, which is many times more potent an agonist (chemical activator) of the CB1 receptor and is used for scientific research. According to Martin Lee, such potent drugs "have been very useful experimentally because they drive the receptor more intensely than do THC or the endocannabinoids. While this property (being a 'high-efficacy full agonist') can create more readily observable results when compared to a partial agonist like THC, such experiments are frequently and inaccurately publicized as revealing a specific effect of marijuana."

In the case of THC, synthetically derived single-molecule pharmaceuticals have been available for the consumer market since 2004. THC-only medicines like Marinol (dronabinol) are pharmaceuticals developed to target specific ailments, like cancer-related nausea. Marinol is synthetically derived THC that is suspended in sesame seed oil, and according to Dr. Ethan Russo, people often discontinue it due to negative side effects. Russo believes this is at least in part because of the absence of other cannabinoids, as reported by *Scientific American* in 2017. "They get anxious, dysphoric, [and] scattered," he says. "It interferes with their ability to function."

Synthetic versions of CBD also exist and are currently used in scientific studies with animal test subjects. There are no FDA-approved single molecule CBD pharmaceuticals available to the consumer market, yet. The data from these animal studies is often hard to compare with an equivalent dose from a CBD-rich extract in humans, meaning our clinical understanding of CBD is still in its infancy. But generally speaking, synthetic cannabinoids are viewed with skepticism by practitioners and patients alike.

As a consumer, one thing to be aware of is that dangerous synthetic and/or counterfeit CBD products have found their

HEALING with CBD

way onto the market. At least 52 people in Utah were sickened by these products between October 2017 and January 2018, according to a report released by the Centers for Disease Control (CDC). Of these 52 people who became ill, 31 ended up in the emergency room with symptoms like altered mental status, seizures, confusion, loss of consciousness, and hallucinations. Brands such as Yolo CBD Oil were being sold as pure CBD, and purchased through smoking and head shops. This underscores the need for consumers to vet their CBD products with lab test results. See Chapter 11: Finding Products You Can Trust for more.

Receptors and Physiology of the ECS

As explained by Martin Lee, "cannabinoid receptors function as subtle sensing devices, tiny vibrating scanners perpetually primed to pick up biochemical cues that flow through fluids surrounding each cell."

As we've mentioned, the ECS is equipped with specialized receptors to pick up cannabinoids (endo-, phyto-, and synthetic varieties). These receptors, called CB1 and CB2 receptors, are located all over the body. Lee continues to explain: "Marijuana does so much and is such a versatile medicine because it acts everywhere, not just in the brain."

The CB1 receptors are most abundant in the central nervous system, connective tissues, glands, and organs like the uterus, cardiovascular system, GI tract, pancreas, bones, and liver, with the brain containing most of these receptors. CB2 receptors are more often found on immune cells, in the gastrointestinal tract, and in the peripheral nervous system.

CB2 receptors are also present in the brain, gut, spleen, liver, heart, kidneys, bones, blood vessels, lymph cells, endocrine glands, and reproductive organs.

Many tissues contain both CB1 and CB2 receptors, where they carry out different actions. Cannabinoid receptors are the most plentiful receptors in the body, more numerous than any other receptor system.

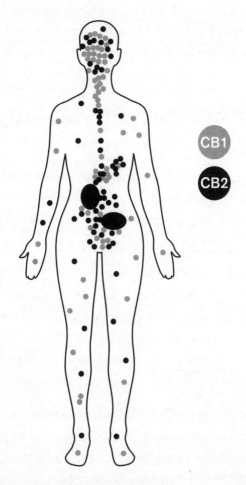

Location of the CB1 and CB2 cannabinoid receptors in the body.

Location of CB1 Receptors in the Brain and Physiological Effects

- Hippocampus: Learning, memory, stress related to memories

- Hypothalamus: Appetite

- Cerebellum: Motor coordination

- Limbic system: Anxiety

- Cerebral cortex: Pain, higher cognitive function

- Nucleus accumbens: Reward and addiction

- Basal ganglia: Sleep and movement

- Medulla: Nausea and vomiting

Our endocannabinoids, anandamide and 2-AG, interact with both receptors; however, anandamide interacts primarily with the CB1 receptors while 2-AG interacts primarily with CB2 receptors.

The list of brain functions that are impacted by the endocannabinoid system is quite long! Decision making, cognition, emotions, learning, memory, regulation of movement, anxiety, stress, fear, appetite, and sense of reward are all affected. When CB1 receptors are activated in the brain, it provides pain and anxiety relief, mood stabilization, and feelings of pleasure and well-being. When CB2 receptors are activated in the brain, it creates a localized anti-inflammatory effect, which is noteworthy because we now know that many neurodegenerative diseases like Alzheimer's and Parkinson's, post-traumatic stress disorder, multiple sclerosis, depression, autoimmune disorders, and cancer have been linked to chronic brain inflammation. The CB2 receptor is also particularly vital to the ECS's ability to generate new nerve cells in the adult brain, crucial to maintaining adult neuroplasticity throughout life.

Outside the brain, anandamide and 2-AG function more as immune system activators than neurotransmitters, focused on stopping inflammation. A 2016 study by K. A. Sharkey and J. W. Wiley concluded that virtually all major GI function is controlled by the ECS. Most of the CB2 receptor actions in the immune system (where they are most plentiful) are involved in reducing inflammation, and tempering immune response, reducing swelling, along with influencing cell migration and programmed cell death.

Cannabis Science Deep Dive

The science behind how cannabis works with our own natural endocannabinoid system is fascinating and complex. Because cannabis has such widespread effects throughout the body at the cellular level, it can provide a level of deep healing that is, according to Martin Lee, "way beyond symptom relief, it's deep healing." For a deep dive on the science of cannabis and CBD, check out Green Flower Media's CBD Summit, an online video resource where Lee explains the mechanisms at work and how cannabis heals at the cellular level.

So in summary, we know that the endocannabinoid system (with the help of cannabinoids and their receptors) impacts:

- Sleep

- Appetite, digestion, hunger

- Mood

- Motor control

- Immune function

- Reproduction and fertility

- Pleasure and reward

- Pain and inflammation

- Memory

- Temperature regulation

- Neurogenesis (growth and development of nervous tissue)

One point to underscore here, as it is underscored in Chapter 9, is that cannabis medicine is not a one-size-fits-all solution: not all the medicinal effects of cannabis are desirable or appropriate for every medical use.

Cannabis and the Opioid Crisis

Cannabis has gained traction as a natural and nonaddictive source of pain relief in the face of a growing opioid crisis. The Centers for Disease Control announced that more than 42,000 people died from opioid overdose in 2016. Within the brain, there are 10 times as many CB1 cannabinoid receptors (which modulate pain response) as there are the "mu" opioid receptors (responsible for the effects of morphine, for example). Research has shown that THC can enhance the efficacy of opioids, meaning that less opioid is needed to provide the same effect. In addition to this, cannabinoids affect the nucleus accumbens region of the brain, which modulates the reward circuit and is involved in addiction. Cannabis has been approved in several state medical programs to treat the symptoms of opioid withdrawal, and research is showing that CBD is particularly effective for this.

Free Radicals and Oxidative Stress

Another important function of the endocannabinoid system is in the scavenging of oxygen **free radicals**. Its effect on scavenging oxygen free radicals is applicable to all disease processes, meaning the ECS holds the keys for understanding and treating the extremely wide and diverse range of human disease.

So, what is a free radical? Free radicals are well-described by Dr. Andrew Weil, a world-renowned leader and pioneer in the field of integrative medicine, on his personal website: they are "electronically unstable atoms or molecules capable of stripping electrons from any other molecules they meet in an effort to achieve stability." Molecules are made up of atoms, and atoms are made up of protons, neutrons, and electrons, which live in a balanced state of neutrality.

Under normal circumstances, every cell in our body produces a certain small amount of oxygen-containing substances, or by-product. This by-product is from the normal cellular processes of our body: reproduction, elimination, growth, nutrition, transport, and syntheses, in addition to the contributions made by external sources like tobacco smoke, pesticides, radiation, industrial toxins, and pollutants. The oxygen created by these natural processes are split into single atoms with unpaired electrons, called free radicals. These unstable free radicals rip through the body trying to find other electrons to pair up with.

These highly reactive radicals can start a chain reaction, like dominoes. Their chief danger comes from the damage they can do when they react with important cellular components such as DNA or the cell membrane. Cells may function poorly or die if this occurs.

When left unchecked and free to develop unhindered, free radicals cause damage that can overwhelm the body. More from Dr. Weil: "By the time a free radical chain fizzles out, it may have ripped through vital components of cells like a tornado, causing extensive damage, similar to that caused by ionizing radiation." This process causes a condition called **oxidative stress,** when the cells' antioxidant system is overwhelmed by the amount of free radicals. The greater the number of free radicals in your body, the more damage is likely to be done. Our bodies work hard to keep these free radicals under control, keeping us in a state of homeostasis.

According to Dr. Joel Fuhrman, board-certified family physician and president of the Nutritional Research Foundation:

*"The body has ways of dealing with oxidative damage;
a potent system of its own antioxidants that scavenge
free radicals or convert them into less dangerous forms,
slowing or stopping the damage. There are also cellular
systems that repair oxidative damage, and others that
induce cell death if there is too much damage."*

Oxidative stress is thought to contribute to bodily aging,
cancer, all inflammatory diseases (arthritis, vasculitis,
glomerulonephritis, lupus erythematous, adult respiratory
diseases syndrome), ischemic diseases (heart diseases, stroke,
intestinal ischemia), acquired immunodeficiency syndrome,
emphysema, gastric ulcers, diabetes, hypertension and
preeclampsia, neurological disorders (Alzheimer's disease,
Parkinson's disease, muscular dystrophy), alcoholism, and
smoking-related diseases, just to name a few.

Understanding the accumulative effects and proper control of
free radicals and oxidative stress, it's no wonder that a search
for nontoxic natural compounds with antioxidative properties
pushes researchers to discover alternatives and ways to
boost our own endogenous system. Instead of management
of symptoms after disease has occurred, with a better
understanding of the endocannabinoid system, we would
hope to prevent disease and cancer by manipulating the ECS.

CHAPTER 4

Cannabinoids and the Entourage Effect

"The number of potential synergies of medicinal interest within the cannabis plant boggles the mind and should keep researchers quite busy for at least the next decade."

—Michael Backes, author of *Cannabis Pharmacy: The Practical Guide to Medical Marijuana*

Most people don't realize that cannabis is chock-full of active compounds, over 400 in fact! Cannabinoids are a big subset of these active compounds, with THC being the best known, and more recently, CBD stealing the spotlight. But there are over 100 other cannabinoids in the cannabis plant that are working behind the scenes of scientific understanding to provide therapeutic benefit: **cannabinol** (CBN), **cannabichromene** (CBC), and **cannabigerol** (CBG), for example.

These cannabinoids offer a veritable treasure trove for our endocannabinoid systems, with more and more research being done to understand their therapeutic potential. In fact, there is initial scientific support for something called "the entourage effect," which we will discuss in detail shortly.

To begin, let's look at a couple of the more popular cannabinoids to garner research attention: tetrahydrocannabinol (THC) and cannabinol (CBN). Cannabidiol (CBD, and don't worry, there won't be a quiz on all the oh-so-similar cannabinoid names) will be covered in its own chapters. In this chapter, we will also cover the relatively new excitement around cannabinoid acids and discuss how the active compounds in cannabis work together to provide some seriously beneficial synergies and a one-two punch known as the entourage effect.

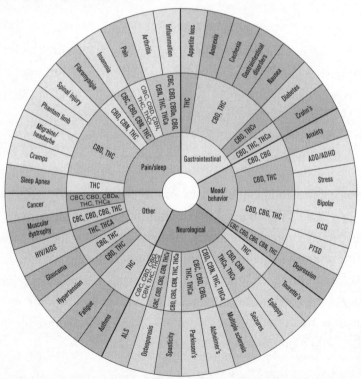

Cannabinoids and the therapeutic effects they can provide.

HEALING with CBD

THC

THC Overview

MEDICINAL USES	PHYSICAL EFFECTS	CONDITIONS TREATED
• Psychoactive • Reduces stress and depression • Appetite stimulant • Dulls pain • Neuroprotectant • Minimizes inflammation • Anti-proliferative (anti-cancer) • Antiemetic (prevents vomiting)	• Euphoria • Relaxation • Giddiness • Introspective dreaminess • Sleepiness • Time distortion • Hunger	• MS • Fibromyalgia • Glaucoma • AIDS • Cancer • PTSD • Spinal injuries • Migraines • Sleep apnea • Insomnia • Anorexia • Crohn's disease • Depression and anxiety • Tourette's syndrome • Epilepsy

Tetrahydrocannabinol, notoriously known for getting people "high," is likely the only cannabinoid most folks are familiar with when it comes to cannabis. While the stigmas associated with THC and cannabis in general continue to linger, an old adage comes to mind: You don't want to throw away the baby with the bathwater. While these stigmas provided the impetus for the bulk of research that was initially done on THC, the happy result is that THC is now the most well-understood of its 100+ brothers and sisters in the plant. While its euphoric effects have been demonized for the better part of this century, the truth of the matter is that this compound is important, some might even say essential, to include in our wellness toolbox.

While THC produces the well-known euphoric effects associated with cannabis, it is equally responsible for the majority of other pharmacological impacts. "Full-spectrum" or "whole-plant" cannabis products usually have a soothing and comforting effect on the mind. Moderate doses tend to induce a sense of well-being and a dreamy state of relaxation. The medicinal benefits of cannabis affect the perception of pain, mood, hunger, and muscle control.

Full-Spectrum, Whole-Plant vs. Isolates

When you hear the term "full-spectrum" or "whole-plant," it typically refers to a plant extract or product that contains all the cannabinoids and other active compounds naturally found in the plant it was taken from. This is to differentiate from CBD- or THC-only products, which are called "isolates." Cannabis or hemp flower is naturally full-spectrum; however, any product made with an extract can be "full-spectrum/whole-plant" or an "isolate," depending on the extraction method and how much the extract has been refined. See Chapter 11: Finding Products You Can Trust for more on extraction methods. The idea of the entourage effect goes hand in hand with that of whole-plant medicine, and you will often hear the two ideas come up together in discussing sources of CBD.

Feeling "high," an idea that has taken on a negative connotation but is only one of the therapeutic effects of THC, is often described as a feeling of euphoria, relaxation, giddiness, introspective dreaminess, sleepiness, and time distortion. The euphoria THC can induce has come to be viewed in a poor light and is the reason many people steer clear of cannabis. To a new cannabis consumer, the feeling can be scary and disorienting, but with the correct doses and an open mind, it can be a therapeutic and life-affirming effect in and of itself, not to mention the medicinal value THC also provides.

THC is known to relieve inflammation and allergic reactions; prevent the nausea, vomiting, and nerve pain associated with cancer medicines; and increase the appetites of people with AIDS. For serious conditions like these, higher levels of THC may be needed to provide patients with relief.

Yet the majority of the patients I speak with state that they don't want to be high. You can indeed use THC and reap all the benefits that this compound has to offer while feeling in control. Understanding what THC can do beyond euphoria or being high will increase the likelihood of having a positive experience if you decide to include this cannabinoid in your wellness plan.

For patients that are new to medical cannabis, THC sensitivity will be higher than those who use cannabis regularly. This doesn't mean that THC needs to be eliminated from treatment! The key with THC, and with any new cannabis product you might be trying for the first time, is to start low and go slow. This is the tried, tested, and true way of titrating (figuring out your ideal dosage, see Chapter 10 for more) with cannabis, and will allow you to find your own individual sweet spot where you can balance psychoactive effects with therapeutic ones in a way that works best for you.

One of the key differences between THC and CBD is that CBD is non-euphoric, meaning that it will not get you high. THC and CBD are found in varying amounts in both types of plants (hemp and cannabis). However, generally speaking, THC is found in much higher proportions in cannabis, and CBD in much higher proportions in hemp.

In fact, THC often dominates the chemical makeup of cannabis, and in recent decades, breeders have worked to increase the amount of THC in strains across the board. Today, strains average in the mid-teens as far as the percentage of THC content, with the strongest strains clocking in the mid to high twenties. Compare this to 40 years ago when the THC content averaged about 5%! But in today's booming cannabis industry, a plethora of products with varying amounts of THC and CBD are available (see Chapter 11: Finding Products You Can Trust).

How THC Works in Your Body

THC binds with the specialized cannabinoid receptors (CB1 and CB2 receptors) that make up the endocannabinoid system. It has a much higher affinity for the CB1 receptors, particularly those in the brain. It works by imitating the effects of anandamide, a neurotransmitter produced naturally in the human brain that modulates sleep, appetite, and pain perception. THC also works with CB2 receptors in the peripheral nervous system, metabolic tissue, and immune system, where it acts as an anti-inflammatory.

According to a 2016 study by C. Walter et al., THC decreases signaling between the sensory part of the brain and the emotional part. This reduces the overall experience of pain by disconnecting the sensation of pain from its emotional impact. This is important because it is the emotional aspects of pain that are tied to a person's sense of self. There is also increasing evidence that THC itself can be an anti-cancer agent by destroying cancer cells, limiting tumor growth, and aiding the body in tumor detection.

Effects and Common Uses

As mentioned, the high associated with cannabis may produce a variety of effects that lead to an altered sense of time and space, enhanced appetite, impaired short-term memory, feelings of happiness, and occasional drowsiness. In low doses, THC has shown promise for its ability to reduce some pain and muscle spasms, stimulate appetite, and help reduce nausea (among many other benefits) with a safety profile that pharmaceuticals can't compete with. Each of these effects vary greatly depending on who is using it, their age, how much they are using, how they are using it, and how often. See Chapter 10: How Much Should I Take for dosing strategies.

Tolerance, Dependence, Addiction, and Overdose

With any psychoactive chemical there is risk of developing a tolerance, dependence, or addiction. For 6% to 9% of the population, THC can become problematic. Most people understand the basic concept of addiction, but what about "tolerance" or "dependence"?

Tolerance

Tolerance is a natural by-product of repeated use and happens with many medications that are taken regularly for long periods of time. Tolerance can happen when the liver becomes more proficient at breaking down and metabolizing the drug (pharmacokinetic tolerance), or because the total number of receptors or the strength of the bond (affinity) between drug and receptor decreases (pharmacodynamic tolerance). So, there are two ways that your body can and does develop a tolerance for cannabis. Tolerance is not the same as dependence or addiction, and tolerance for a drug can increase without dependence or addiction becoming a problem.

Dependence vs. Addiction

Dependence can be either physical or psychological, and it refers to a strong desire to experience the effects of the drug.

Cannabis dependence is generally mild and doesn't produce any major medical or psychiatric issues. It also occurs far less frequently than dependence to alcohol, tobacco, or other drugs. When someone is dependent upon a drug, they may experience cravings to use or mild withdrawal symptoms like irritability, anxiety, or sleeplessness when they stop taking it.

Addiction, on the other hand, is compulsive and overwhelming involvement with a drug. Uncontrollable craving to use grows more important than anything else, including family, friends, career, and even one's own health and happiness. Cannabis does not typically produce this kind of behavior in users, though as mentioned, use may become problematic in 6% to 9% of cannabis users. Comparing cannabis to other drugs like OxyContin (oxycodone), controlled substances with a well-known and very high risk for addiction that are prescribed and used every day, these numbers are relatively small. The overall safety record of cannabis blows drugs like these out of the water.

Overdose

While it is certainly possible to overmedicate and experience very negative side effects with medicines containing THC, it is nearly impossible to induce a lethal overdose with cannabis. The National Cancer Institute states, "Because cannabinoid receptors, unlike opioid receptors, are not located in the brain stem areas controlling respiration, lethal overdoses from cannabis and cannabinoids do not occur."

What to Do If You Overmedicate with THC

Perhaps you've heard a story or have yourself experienced overmedicating with THC. These stories aren't uncommon, and unfortunately, one bad experience with THC can put people off cannabis altogether. This is why you will often hear the advice to "start low and go slow" when it comes to THC, CBD, or any cannabinoid-based medicine! A starting dose of even 1 milligram that is increased slowly over time can allow your body to acclimate to the medicine. But what should you do if you accidentally overmedicate with THC?

The first important point is to try your absolute best to remain calm and know that the experience is not life-threatening (even though it might feel awful) and will be temporary. If you've overmedicated with THC, you might feel nauseous, anxious, and paranoid, along with an increased heart rate. Try to find a quiet and safe space where you can limit stimuli and do some deep breathing. The "4-7-8 technique" (developed by Dr. Andrew Weil) involves breathing in deeply for a count of four, holding your breath for a count of seven, then breathing out slowly for a count of eight. Repeating this several times should soothe the body, mind, and nervous system. Drink plenty of water!

According to Dr. Jordan Tishler, gentle external stimuli like relaxing music, television, or a funny movie can be helpful for getting out of your head. "Over-intoxication tends to make people feel like it will never end. Actively remind yourself that it will end. Try to go to sleep."

You can also try consuming some CBD, which has been shown anecdotally to support countering the negative effects of overmedicating. Scientifically, initial animal studies suggest that CBD might counter the negative psychological effects of THC, though we are yet to see if this translates into humans.[7]

Though CBD may not technically reduce the THC high, its anti-anxiety effects seem to be quite helpful!

Cannabinol (CBN)

CBN Overview

MEDICINAL USES	PHYSICAL EFFECTS	CONDITIONS TREATED
• Analgesic (pain relief) • Sleep aid • Bone growth • Antibacterial • Anti-inflammatory • Anticonvulsant • Appetite stimulant • Antiproliferative	• Relaxation • Sleepiness • Hunger	• Fibromyalgia • Insomnia • Arthritis • Epilepsy/seizures • Multiple sclerosis • Spasticity (tightness, stiffness, or pull of muscles) • Osteoporosis • Amyotrophic lateral sclerosis (ALS) • Psoriasis/eczema • Asthma • Lung cancer

Cannabinol is a cannabinoid found in small quantities in fresh cannabis plants; however, the amount of CBN increases when cannabis is aged and oxidized. It turns out that CBN is actually produced as a by-product when THC breaks down (see

Cannabinoid Acids on page 74). With time and oxygen, THC will convert to CBN. Because quantities of CBN are higher in "old" cannabis plant material, its medicinal properties went mostly unnoticed until recently. But like CBD, cannabinol is being studied as a non-impairing therapeutic aid for people who have sensitivities to or are looking to avoid THC. Now, CBN is being found in cannabis products like topicals, edibles, capsules, and more. In legal and regulated states, CBN content in milligrams should be found on product labeling.

How CBN Works in Your Body

CBN has minimal impact on the central nervous system. Its effects are mainly expressed on a variety of immune cells (T-cells, B-cells, macrophages, and dendritic cells), where CBN has been shown to have strong immunosuppressive and anti-inflammatory properties. CBN may also aid in the natural cycle of cell life/death, while inhibiting the production of a variety of cytokines (a protein that triggers immune and inflammatory responses in the body). Recent research shows that when consumed orally CBN is converted by the liver into a form that better binds to the CB1 receptor, meaning that ingestion is a good way to consume CBN.

Common Effects and Uses

The main benefit of CBN being sold to consumers at the time of this writing is as a sleep aid/sedative. Preliminary studies in rats have shown that CBN acts as an appetite stimulant, which is great news because CBD tends to suppress appetite. It also seems to have powerful anti-inflammatory properties that could be useful in a number of conditions like asthma and arthritis. Its antibacterial properties could be used for any number of applications, and CBN has even successfully killed off methicillin-resistant *Staphylococcus aureus* (MRSA). CBD and THC also successfully killed off the bacteria. Though more research is needed, CBN might also be useful for bone regeneration and in stimulating the production of new stem cells in bone marrow.

Research has shown that CBN stimulates the same nerve pathways in the body as THC. These nerves, the capsaicin-sensitive sensory nerves, are named for their sensitivity to capsaicin, which is the active heat-producing compound in hot peppers. It's often used in infused pain-relief topicals along with CBN and THC. CBN has also been shown to curb the growth of keratinocytes, the type of skin cell that becomes hyperactive and develop scaly growths in conditions like psoriasis and eczema.

Cannabinoid Acids

As the living cannabis plant grows and develops, cannabinoids are naturally present in an acidic form. These cannabinoid acids are the molecular precursors to the more familiar cannabinoids like THC and CBD.

Heating the plant (for example smoking, vaping, or cooking with it) will **decarboxylate** the cannabinoid acids (see What Is Decarboxylation? on page 75), or convert the acids into their more familiar forms: Acids like THCA and CBDA (the "A" is tacked on to identify the acidic form) are converted into the active compounds: THC and CBD, for example. You might hear these two forms of cannabinoids referred to as "acidic cannabinoids" versus "activated cannabinoids." Acidic cannabinoids can also be used by our endocannabinoid systems, and research is suggesting they might be more effective than in their activated forms.

Initial research and anecdotal evidence is suggesting that the acids in their natural state have wonderful therapeutic benefits all on their own, without any euphoria or impairment-inducing effects (like those associated with THC, for example). The bioavailability of cannabinoid acids is an area of debate and inquiry at the time of this writing, where initial research is showing that some cannabinoids, like CBD, might be better absorbed in their acid state and others, like THC, are better absorbed in their activated forms. See page 168 for more on bioavailability.

WHAT IS DECARBOXYLATION?

Decarboxylation refers to the transformation process that cannabinoids go through with the application of heat, and to a lesser extent, time. At the molecular level, when cannabis is heated (smoked, vaped, etc.), the carboxyl group (an acidic group frequently found in biological molecules) on each cannabinoid detaches—it decarboxylates. This causes the cannabinoids to become active. In more simple terms, heat is what makes cannabinoid acids like THCA and CBDA lose their A and become the compounds we're more familiar with, like THC and CBD. Decarboxylation can happen with the passage of time as well, though heating will cause this process to happen instantaneously.

Because acids are most readily available in fresh plant material, unless you live in a state where home-growing is legal, it might be difficult to get a supply of fresh cannabis. Some companies offer tinctures containing cannabinoid acids, but their availability is currently limited to legal states.

Cannabigerolic acid (CBGA) is the "parent" or precursor to other acids like THCA and CBDA. Natural enzymes in cannabis called synthases cause CBGA to break down into THCA and CBDA. On its own, CBGA has been shown to have analgesic (pain relief), antibacterial, and perhaps even antiproliferative (cancer-fighting) properties.

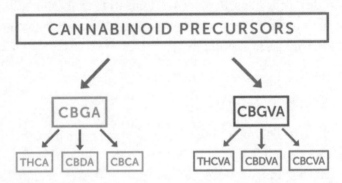

Cannabinoids present in cannabis and hemp plants exist in an acidic and non-impairing form before they are consumed.

THCA, like all cannabinoid acids, is non-impairing. It is, however, being shown to have anti-inflammatory, antiemetic (vomiting), antispasmodic, antiproliferative, and neuroprotective properties. Preliminary research is also showing it might be useful in treating insomnia and used as an appetite stimulant.

While more research is still needed in and around the effects of CBDA, some initial studies have shown it might be helpful in fighting cancer, and it has been shown to inhibit the growth of aggressive breast cancer cells. CBDA might also have anti-inflammatory, antioxidant, and anti-nausea properties.

The Entourage Effect

We are coming to understand, through both preliminary scientific study and a growing tide of anecdotal evidence from patients, that the active compounds in cannabis seem to work together in a very synergistic way, that the whole is bigger than the sum of its parts. According to Dr. John McPartland, "cannabis is inherently polypharmaceutical, and synergy arises from interactions between its multiple components."

Referred to as the entourage effect, this idea is what underlies most conversations you might hear on hemp versus cannabis CBD extracts (see Chapter 7: Sources of CBD: Cannabis and Hemp for more information). Originally proposed by Dr. Raphael Mechoulam and Shimon Ben-Shabat in 1999 and refined by Dr. Ethan Russo in 2010, the main idea behind the entourage effect is that the cannabinoids present in both cannabis and hemp work synergistically together, and synergistically with all the other phytochemicals naturally present in the plants: terpenes, flavonoids, fatty acids, esters, and lactones, for example. Together these compounds can provide a better therapeutic result than any one can on its own. While more research is needed to understand exactly how these complex relationships work, there has been some initial work done examining the synergistic relationship between CBD and THC.

Not only do these active compounds work better together, but the unique way that they come together in any particular **strain** or even an individual plant will determine the therapeutic effect. Breeders have been manipulating genetics for decades to achieve new and unique strains, and this is why you might hear some patients claim that a particular strain might be good for sleep, while another might be better for appetite stimulation. Both hemp and cannabis products can be full-spectrum, meaning they contain CBD and THC in addition to the many other natural compounds (phytochemicals) and phytocannabinoids present in the plant. Where hemp and cannabis products vary is in the volume: how much of each of the cannabinoids and terpenes (among others) they contain.

Hemp-derived extracts, by law, contain minimal amounts of THC (less than 0.3% by dry weight). While they may also contain measurable amounts of other cannabinoids and terpenes, most industrial hemp-derived products will generally contain proportionally less than cannabis-derived products.

A very commonly known example of the entourage effect in action is in the relationship between THC and CBD. THC increases the general efficacy of CBD's therapeutic properties for many people; they work better together. The entourage effect might also explain why synthetic drugs like Marinol (a synthetic THC-isolate) were a flop with patients; see Synthetic Cannabinoids on page 53.

That is not to say that people don't derive benefit from hemp-only derived CBD. Franjo Grotenhermen, former chairman of the International Association for Cannabinoid Medicines, is famously quoted as saying "CBD is CBD" and that our bodies don't care where the molecule comes from. But at this nascent time of CBD science, when patients are really the pioneers of cannabis science and experimentation, the tide of anecdotal evidence seems to be moving toward whole-plant cannabis extracts.

Since the idea was first put forth, studies have helped us understand that different phytocannabinoids can achieve similar outcomes (pain relief, appetite stimulation, or relaxation, as examples), but may achieve them in different ways from one another. This means cannabis can act in a very robust way to provide its therapeutic benefit. Researcher Elisabeth Williamson put it well when she described the synergies among phytochemicals as an "herbal shotgun" as opposed to the "magic bullet" people assume single molecule formulations can provide.[8]

A study in multiple sclerosis patients has shown that a 1:1 ratio of CBD:THC was more effective than pure CBD or pure THC for spasticity. A 2015 study conducted in Israel (which you might remember from Chapter 2 is fast becoming the epicenter in scientific research on cannabis) showed that CBD-rich, whole-plant extracts with low levels of THC, cannabichromene (CBC), cannabigirol (CBG), cannabinol (CBN), and **cannabidivarin** (CBDV) was much more effective for pain relief and as an anti-inflammatory than CBD alone. They also found that the whole-plant medicine had a much wider range for a therapeutic dosage, where CBD-only medicines had a relatively small dosage range where it provided relief. In another study, it was shown that CBD, CBDA, THCA, CBN, and CBG all block prostate cells from growing rapidly. And while pain relief is often associated with THC and CBD, cannabichromene (CBC) also acts as pain reliever by blocking the release of pain neurotransmitters and receptors.

Terpenes

Terpenes are the natural oils that give cannabis, and many other herbs, fruits, and plants, their aroma, color, and flavor.

These distinctive flavors and scents are prized by cannabis enthusiasts and often help identify strains, and even name them: Lemon Haze, Strawberry Cough, or Mango Tango, for example. They have also given the plant a huge evolutionary advantage by helping keep away insects and animal predators, and acting as an antifungal. Terpenes are secreted by the glandular hairs (trichomes) found most densely on the flower leaves and buds of the plant.

Recently terpenes have garnered scientific attention for their synergistic ability to work with cannabinoids and have been identified as heavy hitters in the entourage effect. Terpenes interact with the endocannabinoid system in a similar way to cannabinoids. When inhaled or ingested, the terpenes act as an assistant to cannabinoids as they work to penetrate the blood-brain barrier. Myrcene, for example, is known to increase cell permeability, allowing for faster absorption of THC and other cannabinoids. Terpenes can also influence neurotransmitters in the brain, affecting dopamine and serotonin production and destruction. This insight also gives us an idea as to why different strains not only smell and taste different, but also have varying effects on our mood and physical experience.

Dr. Ethan Russo published a report in 2011 that claims cannabinoid-terpenoid interactions "could produce synergy with respect to treatment of pain, inflammation, depression, anxiety, addiction, epilepsy, cancer, fungal, and bacterial infections."

Most Common Terpenes in Cannabis

	Boiling points	Aromas	Effects	Also found in	Medical benefits
MYRCENE	168°C (334°F)	musk, cloves, herbal, citrus	sedating, relaxing; enhances the THC's psychoactivity	mango, thyme, citrus, lemongrass, bay leaves	antiseptic, anti-bacterial, antifungal, inflammation
CARYOPHYLLENE	160°C (320°F)	pepper, wood, spice	no detectable physical effects	pepper, cloves, hops, basil, oregano	antioxidant, inflammation, muscle spasms, pain, insomnia
LINALOOL	198°C (388°F)	floral, citrus, spice	sedating, calming	lavendar, citrus, laurel, birch, rosewood	insomnia, stress, depression, anxiety, pain, convulsions
PINENE	155°C (311°F)	sharp, sweet, pine	memory retention, alertness	pine needles, conifers, sage	inflammation, asthma (bronchodilator)
HUMULENE	198°C (388°F)	woody, earthy	suppresses appetite	hops, coriander	anti-inflammatory, anti-bacterial, pain
LIMONENE	176°C (349°F)	citrus, lemon, orange	elevated mood, stress relief	citrus rinds, juniper, peppermint	anti-depression, anti-anxiety, gastric reflux, antifungal

Data courtesy of Leafly.com.

Fun fact: All cannabinoids are technically **terpenoids** (terpenes), but they are specific to the cannabis plant! So when we talk about terpenes, we are talking about the more common terpenes also found in herbs, fruits, and other plants. Aside from working synergistically with other compounds in cannabis, terpenes also have health benefits and therapeutic properties all of their own.

Some of the most well-known terpenes and their benefits include:

Humulene is a terpene also found in hops and coriander. It imparts a woody and earthy aroma and flavor to cannabis, and is known to have anti-inflammatory, antibacterial, and pain-relief benefits. It can also act as an appetite suppressant.

Pinene (Alpha and Beta) is a sharp, sweet, and piney-smelling terpene that is also found in pine cones and needles, conifers, rosemary, and sage. It is known to act as a bronchodilator, and has cancer-fighting and anti-inflammatory capabilities. It crosses the blood-brain barrier easily, where it prevents the destruction of molecules that aid memory along with alertness. It can also be used as a local antiseptic.

Linalool is largely responsible for the characteristic soothing smell of lavender. It is also found in citrus, laurel, birch, and rosewood. Linalool offers great sedative benefits, along with being an antiseptic and pain reliever. It activates immune cells and generally boosts the immune system. It can act as an anti-inflammatory, and in 2016 was shown to reverse the effects of Alzheimer's in mice.[9]

Beta-Caryophyllene is a peppery- and spicy-smelling terpene found in black pepper, hops, cloves, basil, and oregano. It is known to be an antioxidant while being anti-inflammatory and offering relief from muscle spasms. A 2014 study[10] showed potential for beta-caryophyllene as a treatment for chronic pain, and it has also been shown to have anti-anxiety and antidepressant effects.[11] It is the only terpene known to

HEALING with CBD

directly activate our cannabinoid receptors (CB2), plus it's the reason leafy greens are so healthy for you!

Myrcene is a musky and citrusy terpene found in mango, thyme, lemongrass, and bay leaves. It is the most common terpene in cannabis and is known to have sedative[12] and analgesic effects.[13] It offers synergistic effects by lowering the blood-brain barrier for itself and other compounds.

Limonene is the bright clean terpene we most associate with citrus fruits but is also found in other plants like juniper and peppermint. It's been known to relieve symptoms of depression and anxiety,[14] and aids in the absorption of other terpenes through the skin and into body tissue.[15] Limonene has antifungal properties, combats gastric reflux,[16] and has shown promise in shrinking cancerous tumors.[17]

Terpineol has refreshing floral, citrus, and spice aromas, and is found naturally in lilacs. It has the ability to reduce pain and inflammation,[18] and can help protect the stomach from ulcers.[19] Used topically it has antibacterial and antimicrobial effects.[20] But it's perhaps best known for its antiproliferative benefits, specifically in targeting tumors.[21]

If you are looking for particular terpenes in products, keep in mind that each state has its own requirements for testing products. Also, as a plant, each season and harvest can vary. The only way to be sure of what you are getting, and in what quantities, is by finding lab-tested products.

If you are using a particular product that has a verified cannabinoid profile, you may notice changes in how the medicine affects you from batch to batch. Eileen has known of children who suffer from Dravet syndrome losing seizure control because of the changes that occur from batch to batch of high-CBD medicines. Reputable companies should be happy to supply you with test results. Not all companies test for all compounds—so be sure to ask!

CHAPTER 5

WHAT IS CANNABIDIOL (CBD)?

"The growing body of science and research supporting CBD as a valid medicine with an extraordinary range of potential applications can simply no longer be ignored."

—Leonard Leinow in *CBD: A Patient's Guide to Medical Cannabis*

You probably picked up this book because you are curious about cannabidiol (pronounced ka-nah-beh-die-all). Whether you want to understand why this ingredient is popping up everywhere, or you are suffering from a particular ailment or disease and you've heard CBD might help, you have come to the right place!

If you're a real go-getter and you dived directly into this chapter, you'll get a good overview as to what CBD is and how it works in your body. The next chapter will discuss the two main sources of CBD: hemp and cannabis. Chapter 8 will cover what conditions and symptoms CBD can be helpful in treating, while the rest of the book offers a practical guide on how to use CBD products, how much to take, and how to evaluate the quality and safety of various products. You can use the preceding chapters of this book to fill in any holes as you go along on your journey.

There is no doubt that CBD is the cannabis medicinal *du jour*: CBD is being added to everything from coffee beans to bottled water, gummies to make-up! The excitement around the health benefits of CBD is certainly not going unnoticed by entrepreneurs and manufacturers.

This explosion in the consumer products market is being driven by CBD's incredible potential as a healing and therapeutic agent. The forefront of CBD science is an exciting place! And CBD has become a hot topic in treating childhood epilepsy and traumatic brain injuries in athletes. It's also an area of keen interest in the veterinary world. (Yes, CBD can help not just your pets, but countless animals. See What CBD Can Do for Your Pets on page 156 for more information.)

Unfortunately, among all this excitement there is also a lot of misinformation and a general lack of understanding as to what CBD is and how it can be used. An unfortunate by-product of 80+ years of cannabis and hemp prohibition is that there are no solid regulatory frameworks in place at the federal level to protect consumers, and you can be sure that not all CBD products are created equally. All this leads to a lot of confusion around cannabidiol.

So let's start with the basics.

Cannabidiol: The Big Picture

CBD has been in the public spotlight since around 2012, although scientists have been aware of its potential for over a decade. It was in the early part of the 2000s when CBD's true potential began to shine: Its remarkable versatility and synergy with THC was finally recognized, along with a growing understanding that there is a synergistic relationship between all the different compounds developed on the plant (see Chapter 4: Cannabinoids and The Entourage Effect).

CBD has a very wide spectrum of potential therapeutic benefits. As a single compound, it offers a large number of treatment options for an astoundingly large variety of seemingly unrelated diseases and conditions, and we will shed a little light on how and why that is in this chapter. But in the big-picture sense, CBD has significant and profound effects on how our body maintains balance in the face of countless external stressors. Its reach is wide and deep: CBD works seamlessly with our own natural bodily systems, producing its effects at the molecular level and going far beyond symptom relief to actually helping our body heal itself, all the while producing no impairment whatsoever.

WOW, right? The more we learn about CBD, the more it seems poised to revolutionize medicine as we know it.

So it's easy to see why CBD has gained such popularity: CBD works with our bodies in such a way as to legitimately be able to treat a wide variety of conditions AND it lacks the impairment associated with THC. The impairment piece is important to a lot of people. There is still stigma around getting high, and it's legitimately an unpleasant or undesirable experience for many patients. Even if you're not opposed to the pyschotropic effects of THC (see Is Getting High Bad for You? on page 94), CBD can provide relief during the course of the day when you probably need a clear head for work and daily life.

Our society can become healthier as more energy and resources are being put into research focused on uncovering the synergies of the different compounds of cannabis and their complementary roles in helping with pain, cancer, mind disorders, and many other chronic debilitating conditions. Destigmatizing cannabis, both in the minds of the general public and our politicians, is essential because these stigmas prevent many from looking at the vast potential of cannabis-based medicines as viable options/additions or alternative treatments in their lives.

CBD is the most abundant nonintoxicating compound found in cannabis and hemp. There are over 400 active compounds developed in the plant; phytocannabinoids (aka cannabinoids), terpenoids (aka terpenes), and flavonoids are but a few that have garnered our attention. It is the diversity and concentration of these compounds that compels some scientists to refer to cannabis as a "pharmacological treasure trove" of potential. These active compounds are found in an oily resin that is developed within the trichomes (tiny hairs) of the plant. Not only that, but many of these compounds (called cannabinoids) are unique to cannabis and hemp.

Yes, you read that right. Hemp is part of the CBD conversation, and becoming an increasingly big part of it as demand for CBD in the consumer market grows.

HEALING with CBD

CBD in a Nutshell

- The active compounds in hemp and cannabis are called "cannabinoids."

- CBD is a cannabinoid.

- Human beings, and many living creatures, have natural bodily systems that use CBD.

- The endocannabinoid system (ECS) is the primary system that uses CBD.

- CBD is non-euphoric.

How It Works

The main benefit CBD confers to humans (and many other creatures, too) is as an anti-inflammatory agent. We are coming to appreciate that inflammation is the common seed for many forms of disease and underlies seemingly unrelated conditions like Alzheimer's disease and cancer. CBD acts to reduce or prevent inflammation in both the brain and body, and this simple action can have huge impacts on your health and well-being.

So how does CBD do it?

CBD works in our bodies through the endocannabinoid system, a master regulatory mechanism for the entire body. (See Chapter 3: The Endocannabinoid System.)

CBD in the Brain and Body

CBD impacts our bodies by working indirectly on both the CB1 and CB2 receptors, stimulating these receptors while also blocking a key enzyme from breaking down our own endogenous cannabinoid anandamide, effectively making CBD a reuptake and breakdown inhibitor. This increases the levels of anandamide in the brain and is thought to be why CBD has proven to be so effective at helping to manage seizures. By acting as a reuptake inhibitor (preventing the reabsorption) for the neurotransmitter adenosine, CBD is able to provide anti-anxiety and anti-inflammatory effects.

Another way CBD provides therapeutic effect is by binding to several non-cannabinoid receptors in the brain.

By directly stimulating the serotonin 5HT1A receptor, CBD can impact anxiety, appetite, sleep, perception of pain, mood, nausea and vomiting, and sexual behavior, to name a few. New science is showing that CBDA (the acidic form of CBD in raw plants, see page 74 for more information) also has a high affinity for the 5-HT1A serotonin receptor, and is proving to have even more powerful anti-nausea effects than CBD and THC. CBD also interacts directly with the TRPV1 receptor, which is known to mediate pain perception, inflammation, and body temperature. Our own endogenous anandamide also stimulates the TRPV1 receptor.

CBD blocks the GPR55 receptor, and by doing so can both help prevent osteoporosis and limit cancer cell proliferation. By stimulating the PPAR-gamma receptor, CBD can also have an antiproliferative effect as well as limit tumor growth in human lung cancer. PPAR-gamma activation can also help degrade the amyloid-beta plaque associated with Alzheimer's. And if that wasn't enough, PPAR receptors also regulate genes that are involved in energy homeostasis, lipid uptake, insulin sensitivity, and other metabolic functions. Because of its influence on PPAR receptors, CBD might be a future treatment option for diabetes and other metabolic dysfunctions.

It is primarily through its work on all these receptors that CBD provides an impressive array of therapeutic benefits, benefits that go way beyond symptom relief to provide deep healing at the molecular level. Just check out the list of CBD's major medicinal properties! Research in all these areas will continue to refine our understanding of CBD and the ECS as a whole, and will no doubt uncover more new and exciting applications for CBD.

Major Medicinal Properties of CBD

The major medicinal effects of CBD that are currently being investigated include:

• Antiemetic: Combats nausea and vomiting

• Anticonvulsant: Combats seizure activity

• Antipsychotic: Combats psychosis disorders

• Anti-inflammatory: Combats inflammatory disorders

• Antioxidant: Combats neurodegenerative disorders

• Antitumoral/Anticancer: Combats tumor and cancer cells

• Anxiolytic (anti-anxiety)/Antidepressant: Combats anxiety and depression disorders

See Chapter 8 for more detail on CBD's medicinal properties.

Let's address one more major way in which CBD, and all cannabinoids, provide us with some serious health advantages. Phytocannabinoids have both antioxidant and neuroprotective properties, and potent ones at that.

You may have heard that antioxidants are important, but you might not realize just how important they are. Our bodies produce antioxidants but not nearly enough to counteract the amount of oxidative stress that is thrown our way in everyday modern life. Diets rich in antioxidants have been shown to reduce the risk of diseases like cardiovascular disease, stroke, Parkinson's disease, Alzheimer's disease, and arthritis. The National Cancer Institute recognizes the therapeutic potential of antioxidants for preventing the types of free radical damage that have been associated with cancer. A study published in 1998 was one of the first to document CBD's antioxidant properties, and CBD was found to be a more powerful antioxidant than both vitamins C and E![22]

Neuroprotectants protect, not surprisingly, our brains. As a neuroprotectant, CBD helps reduce damage to the brain and nervous system and encourages the growth and development of new neurons. Oxidative stress caused by ischemia (inadequate blood supply), traumatic blows, or autoimmune and genetic disorders can cause temporary or permanent neural damage, but studies have shown that CBD is able to protect against this damage and improve recovery.

These findings suggest that CBD could be therapeutically beneficial for traumatic brain injuries, spinal cord injuries, spinal cord diseases, and strokes. CBD's neuroprotective properties are also potentially beneficial in helping prevent and limit the progression of neurological disorders, such as ALS, epilepsy, MS, and Parkinson's disease. More research to investigate CBD's efficacy for promoting cell and neuron health are needed, but the evidence so far suggests that CBD could be used to minimize neural and cell damage and encourage healing.

CBD Doesn't Get You High

One of the most highly touted benefits of CBD is the fact that it won't get you high. As we've mentioned, this point is very important to a lot of people and makes CBD an attractive treatment option for people who cannot tolerate THC as part of their treatment.

This lack of euphoria has many in the public mislabeling CBD as non-psychoactive, which just isn't the case. So let's refine this idea a little bit, because while CBD won't get you high, to say that it's not "psychoactive" isn't entirely accurate. According to Dr. Ethan Russo, "...these terms (non-psychotropic/non-psychoactive) are inaccurate given its (CBD's) prominent pharmacological benefits on anxiety, schizophrenia, addiction, and possibly even depression."

A quick search in the Merriam-Webster dictionary:

Psychoactive: Affecting the mind or behavior

Psychotropic: Acting on the mind

Cannabidiol clearly has an effect on the mind; it's one of its most prized effects. Just because something acts on your brain does not mean that it's a negative thing. And acting on the mind doesn't automatically mean it will get you high. Lots of pharmaceuticals (antidepressants for example) act on the mind and don't get you high!

But is "getting high" that big a deal? Is getting tipsy that big a deal? You'd probably say "no" to getting tipsy, but there is still stigma around the euphoric effects of THC. And yet, waking up after a night of consuming cannabis feels nothing like waking up after a night of drinking.

Of course, the nonintoxicating effects of CBD are extremely beneficial, and the fact that CBD doesn't make you high gives it more versatility than high-THC treatment options. To be clear: We are not here to propose that the euphoric effects of THC are the right thing for everyone. But we are here to challenge the stigma around the euphoric effects of THC because not only can THC make you feel good, but it can also provide therapeutic benefit in the process.

Is Getting High Bad for You?

The idea that using medication to feel good isn't appropriate or acceptable seems to almost uniquely apply to cannabis. Tranquilizers and antidepressants, for example, are intended to make us feel emotionally better. Of course, the euphoria associated with THC might be totally off the table and undesirable for some people, and won't be useful or appropriate in certain situations. But the experience of laughing, enjoying food, music, and the people around you more, feeling the spark of creativity, feeling more open-minded and patient—these effects can be as therapeutic as pain relief and reduced inflammation. Famed cannabis activist and advocate Steve DeAngelo often refers to these as the "overlooked wellness benefits" of cannabis.

Besides, THC and CBD share a special symbiotic relationship. They both offer potent anti-inflammation and analgesic effects but do so through different mechanisms in the body and brain. This means a more robust overall effect. CBD also prolongs the therapeutic effects of THC by delaying its breakdown by the body. Through new studies on the science of the entourage effect coupled with countless patient stories, CBD often works better with THC. In this exciting new age of cannabis therapeutics, you can reap the benefits of THC without any of the euphoric effects. The takeaway: if you live in a state where it's available to you, don't be afraid to experiment with THC in your medicine!

CHAPTER 6

Is CBD Safe?

"Marijuana in its natural form is one of the safest therapeutically active substances known to man. By any measure of rational analysis marijuana can be safely used within the supervised routine of medical care."

—Francis L. Young at the 1988 ruling in the matter of "Marijuana Rescheduling Petition"

Is CBD safe? The answer to that is yes! Aside from the long list of medical applications and conditions CBD can help treat, another reason CBD has proven to be so powerful in the medical arena is that it is very safe.

Studies and scientific reviews confirm CBD's safety: In a 2017 review, CBD's safety profile was confirmed and even expanded.[23] Not only that, but CBD was confirmed by the World Health Organization (WHO) in a 2017 report to pose no public health risk or potential for abuse. The WHO report deemed CBD to be very safe and well-tolerated across a wide spectrum of dosages. In 2011, a review found that long-term doses of up to 1,500 milligrams per day were well-tolerated in humans.[24]

In 2018, a WHO committee called for more scientific evidence and further review of CBD in response to the increase in interest from Member States in the use of cannabis for medical indications, including for palliative care, or specialized medical care for people with life-limiting illness. To that end, the Expert Committee on Drug Dependence (ECDD) did an initial review of CBD, and concluded:

> *"Recent evidence from animal and human studies shows that its use could have some therapeutic value for seizures due to epilepsy and related conditions. Current evidence also shows that cannabidiol is not likely to be abused or create dependence as for other cannabinoids (such as tetrahydrocannabinol (THC), for instance). The ECDD, therefore, concluded that current information does not justify scheduling of cannabidiol and postponed a fuller review of cannabidiol preparations to May 2018, when the committee will undertake a comprehensive review of cannabis and cannabis-related substances."*

Despite the intention to conduct a comprehensive review, when the ECDD met in June 2018 they conducted a more limited "pre-review." The results of the pre-review were favorable, concluding that cannabis has therapeutic potential for conditions like chronic pain, appetite stimulation, epilepsy, opioid withdrawal, PTSD, and sleep disorders. They underscored that more robust clinical research and evidence is needed before they make a final determination on the efficacy of cannabis therapeutics for these conditions. They will submit the findings of their pre-review to the WHO, along with a recommendation that an in-depth review be carried out.

Cannabidiol's nonaddictive properties are particularly provocative when considering the severe side effects and high rates of abuse with other prescription drugs, particularly opioids. According to the CDC, there were 32,445 opioid overdose deaths in America in 2016, about 89 per day. The National Cancer Institute states, "Because cannabinoid receptors, unlike opioid receptors, are not located in the brain stem areas controlling respiration, lethal overdoses from cannabis and cannabinoids do not occur."

Another plus for cannabis therapeutics, and where CBD really shines, is in its ability to deliver a one-two punch when it comes to opioid use: not only can CBD treat pain, but it might also help lessen the cravings for and withdrawal symptoms associated with opioid addiction (see Addiction on page 121 for more information).

Cannabis and opioids are "co-agonists," meaning they enhance each other's effectiveness, and many people using cannabis in conjunction with opioids are either able to reduce their dosages or replace the opioids altogether. A survey of 984 patients who use opioids states, "97% percent of the sample 'strongly agreed/agreed' that they are able to decrease the amount of opiates they consume when they also use cannabis, and 81% 'strongly agreed/agreed' that taking cannabis by itself was more effective at treating their condition than taking cannabis with opioids. Results were similar for those using cannabis with nonopioid-based pain medications."[25]

In a 2016 survey of opioid users with chronic pain, 64% reported a decreased use of opioids when adding cannabis to their treatment regimen.[26] A first-of-its-kind, 18-month study will examine whether cannabis decreases the use of opioids in patients suffering from chronic pain at New York's Albert Einstein College of Medicine, while a recent animal study showed that rats treated with CBD gel were less likely to relapse to opioid use.[27]

CBD is already being used to enhance the effects of antiepileptic drugs, often decreasing the dosage (along with reducing unpleasant side effects) or replacing them altogether. In the future, CBD might also become a useful addition to treatment regimens including prescription medications like antidepressant, antipsychotic, and anti-anxiety drugs.

The science supporting CBD has been widely accepted: CBD is safe and well-tolerated. It is all-natural, nontoxic, and non-addictive, and when compared to the side effects and safety profiles of traditional prescription medications, it's no contest.

But other adverse effects (or no effects at all) can arise when it comes to the source, extraction methods, and manufacturing of CBD products (see Chapter 11: Finding Products You Can Trust for more on sourcing high-quality CBD).

Possible Side Effects

While there hasn't been a lot of scientific study looking at the side effects of CBD, we do know for sure that impairment is definitely not one. In fact, studies show that CBD produces no impairment even at very high doses.

A 2017 scientific review shows that most clinical studies have focused on CBD treatment for epilepsy and psychotic disorders, and in these areas, the most common patient side effects included tiredness, diarrhea, and changes of appetite/weight.[28]

Anecdotally, the most common side effects patients report include dizziness, lethargy, sleepiness, hyperactivity, loose stools, jitteriness, and an increased heart rate. Less commonly reported side effects include irritability, increased seizure activity, decreased appetite, alertness, heart palpitations, and insomnia. Minor side effects like headache have also often been reported in conjunction with poor quality CBD oil tinctures.

Drug Interactions

If you want to start taking CBD but you're also taking other prescription medications, you should be aware that there is a chance for drug interaction.

There is a family of liver enzymes, called the cytochrome P450 group, that works to metabolize roughly 60% of the pharmaceutical drugs we consume. At high enough doses, CBD inhibits the activity of these enzymes, which will increase the duration of action and effect of prescription drugs metabolized by the P450 group. Unfortunately, because of the individuality of each person's endocannabinoid system and because each drug seems to have its own unique threshold for CBD sensitivity, there is no standard cut-off dose to avoid this interaction, meaning you will need to work with a doctor to monitor the blood levels of your medications while taking CBD.

If you want to try CBD with other prescription medications, be sure to talk to your doctor or pharmacist. A simple way of determining if you should be concerned about possible CBD interactions is to ask your doctor or pharmacist whether you should avoid eating grapefruit while taking the medication in question. CBD interacts with medications in the same way grapefruit does, only it has much more potent effects. So if the answer is yes, you will know interaction could be an issue for you.

Here are types of drugs that use the cytochrome P450 enzyme system and can interact with CBD:

- Steroids

- HMG-CoA reductase inhibitors

- Calcium channel blockers

- Antihistamines

- Prokinetics

- HIV antivirals

- Immune modulators

- Benzodiazepines

- Antiarrythmics

- Antibiotics

- Anesthetics

- Antipsychotics

- Antidepressants

- Antiepileptics

- Beta blockers

- Proton pump inhibitors (PPIs)

- Nonsteroidal anti-inflammatory drugs (NSAIDs)

- Angiotensin II blockers

- Oral hypoglycemic agents

- Sulfonylureas

If your doctor can't advise you on taking CBD along with your prescription medications, seek out the advice of a licensed cannabis doctor or nurse. See the Resources on page 247 for information on finding one.

CHAPTER 7

Sources of CBD: Cannabis and Hemp

"The key difference between hemp plants and cannabis plants is resin content. Most hemp plants are low-resin plants. Cannabis plants are high-resin plants."

—Martin Lee, author and cofounder of Project CBD

Did you know that CBD can come from both industrial hemp and cannabis? Both plants, though part of the same family, are genetically distinct entities with drastically different pasts and evolutionary paths. They both contain CBD but are markedly different plants in their cultivation, ability to produce CBD, and general application.

There have been real and important legal gains for hemp farming in America in just the last decade or so, with industrial hemp farming resuming for the first time in 80 years. There is a lot of debate around hemp versus cannabis sources of CBD, and there is no clear right or wrong. Not only that, but the whole topic takes on a layer of complexity and confusion given the legal morass that hemp and cannabis currently wade around in. Because while people might think (and producers will often tell you) that hemp-derived CBD is legal, the reality is not so clear-cut.

In this new age of *Cannabis sativa* (referring to the larger taxonomic species that includes both plants) therapeutics, the genetic paths of hemp and cannabis are converging. We are cross-breeding and manipulating genes to offer a plethora of CBD-dominant products to patients, and the lines between hemp and cannabis are blurring. But for the moment, it's still worth talking about these two sources of CBD as being distinctly different.

Can we get controversial for a minute here? We have to when it comes to talking about hemp versus cannabis sources of CBD, because it is a HOT debate right now. Let's begin with some key differences between the plants.

Hemp vs. Cannabis: The Plants

Both cannabis and hemp are members of the same species, *Cannabis sativa*, which is one of humanity's oldest domesticated crops. Throughout history, we have grown different varieties of *Cannabis sativa* for different purposes. Over thousands of years of genetic selection for function, coupled with varying growing environments, two distinct plants have emerged that are very different in their cultivation and use.

Tall, sturdy plants were grown by early civilizations to make a variety of clothing, rope, sails, and building materials. These plants were bred with other plants of similar characteristics, leading to the type of cannabis we now know as hemp. Today hemp plants are grown predominantly for their fiber while others are grown primarily for their seeds to produce oil. We use industrial hemp in a very large number of applications, from car parts to cooking oils, clothing to body creams.

Meanwhile in different parts of the world, other *Cannabis sativa* plants became popular for medicinal and religious purposes, and eventually these plants were bred for their resinous trichomes (more on that later). This led to the unique varieties we now use for medicinal, spiritual, and recreational purposes. Today, medicinal cannabis plants consist of more euphoric THC-rich varieties, non-euphoric CBD-rich varieties, and points in between. In this book, we refer to these plants as simply "cannabis."

WHAT'S IN A NAME?

Throughout this book, we refer to the plant you might know as "marijuana," "weed," or "pot" as simply "cannabis," which is the proper name of the plant. We refrain from using the name "marijuana" because it is historically and racially charged. Hemp is a common and acceptable name for this distinct cousin of cannabis, and useful for distinguishing the two *Cannabis sativa* plants in discussion.

Cannabis sativa, regardless of whether it is a fiber or seed plant (hemp) or a medicinal plant (cannabis), all have the same structural features: stems, stalks, roots, flowers, and leaves.

HEALING with CBD

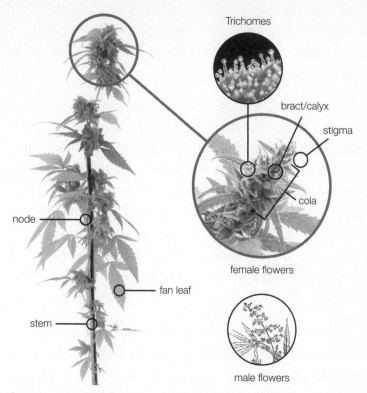

The basic anatomy of the cannabis plant. Hemp plant anatomy, while not exactly the same, is very similar.

Cannabis plants vary in height from 3 to 15 feet tall and have multiple branches with five to seven delicate serrated leaves spread like the fingers of an open hand. The plant's leaves and flowers are covered, as is the entire plant, with tiny sticky hairs. These hairs, like the hairs on so many other plant species, are almost microscopic spikes that develop on the plant's skin.

The technical term for these plant hairs is **trichomes**, and it's a term you will hear a lot in reference to cannabis because these trichomes are where almost all the good stuff is stored. Trichomes may resemble hair, but they're not the same as our hair or the hair on your dog. Trichomes are living cells. They run the gamut in how they look and feel and get classified as either simple or glandular. Glandular trichomes, the ones found on cannabis and hemp, produce and store oils on the plant's surface.

All *Cannabis sativa* plants (hemp and cannabis) develop glandular trichomes. Just as mammal hair serves various protective purposes, including insulation and camouflage, so do trichomes. Trichomes provide a protective layer to the leaves and flowers from frost and UV rays. They also help reduce evaporation by protecting the plant from wind and heat. In many cases, trichomes protect plants from insects as well, with some structures so stiff or irritating (Stinging Nettle, for example) that they can keeps even large herbivores away.

In these trichomes, there is an oily resin of biologically active phytochemicals produced by plants: flavonoids, terpenoids, phenolic compounds, and cannabinoids, among others.

Some phytochemicals (flavonoids) give plants their pretty colors, like the blue in blueberries and the red in raspberries; other phytochemicals (terpenes) give plants their distinctive aromas, like basil, sage, and rosemary. The **phenolic compounds** found in cannabis trichomes have antioxidant properties, an essential component of a healthy diet.

There are lots of different phytochemicals in all the plant foods you eat, and some sources consider them to be nutrients. However, unlike vitamins and minerals, they're not found to be essential nutrients, and there aren't any established dietary reference intakes. Phytochemicals, like the active compounds in echinacea, for example, are extracted from plants, processed, and sold as dietary supplements. They're generally considered to be safe, but there's not much regulation regarding their dosages or even effectiveness.

Cannabinoids are the phytochemicals most people know of in cannabis: THC, for example, and CBD. More specifically, they are referred to phytocannabinoids, meaning they come from plants, unlike the endogenous cannabinoids (anadamide and 2-AG) that our bodies naturally produce.

As the plant grows and develops, the chemical composition of the trichomes changes dramatically. The "chemical cocktail" found within the trichomes of each strain has a different therapeutic effect that is unique to that strain, and even to that plant. There are many factors that contribute to the final chemical makeup of the plant: genetics, where it is grown (indoor, outdoor, greenhouse), what it is fed, when and how it is harvested, and how it is cured, to name but a few. Both cannabis and hemp plants develop these trichomes; however, because historically cannabis has been cultivated for medicinal and recreational use, it's been bred to maximize the development of trichomes. This makes cannabis a much richer source of phytochemicals and cannabinoids.

Industrial hemp plants are genetically predisposed to grow tall and lanky with small flowers, using much of its energy for developing fibers. Medicinal cannabis plants, on the other hand, are designed for phytochemical production, growing shorter and bushier, with more branches that support more flowers and therefore an abundance of therapeutic compounds.

On cannabis, trichomes (and all the good phytochemicals that are stored in their resin) form in abundance on the flowers and upper leaves of female plants, and to a lesser extent on the lower leaves, branches, and stems. Male plants also develop trichomes but far less than the female plants, which is why cannabis growers focus on female plants almost exclusively.

Another useful way to think about the hemp versus cannabis distinction, according to Martin Lee, is in resin content. Generally speaking, hemp plants are low in this phytochemical-rich oil, and cannabis plants are high-resin plants.

As mentioned earlier, historically cannabis cultivation has focused on developing and maximizing trichome production, largely for THC content and the terpenes that give each varietal strain its particular character. Perhaps you've heard of some of the more famous strains like Maui Wowie, Lemon Haze, and Blue Dream. Today, with our improved understanding of CBD and all its therapeutic properties, many cannabis producers have begun to focus on CBD-rich plants. There are several cannabis plants whose primary cannabinoid is CBD, with very low levels of THC.

In its cocktail of cannabinoids, there is proportionally more CBD in hemp than in cannabis: Hemp naturally produces a higher proportion of CBD as compared to other phytocannabinoids, like THC. You can think of it as a pie chart of phytocannabinoids, where in hemp's pie chart, the CBD slice is bigger than in cannabis's. This is one of the reasons that hemp has become such a popular source of CBD and has in turn led to an industrial hemp farming revival here in the US after decades of prohibition. That said, because hemp doesn't naturally produce much in the way of trichomes (as compared to cannabis), it takes far more hemp to get

HEALING WITH CBD

an equivalent amount of CBD. In other words, the cannabis phytocannabinoid pie is just bigger than hemp's. This presents a solid argument as to why CBD extraction might not be the best use of hemp, especially considering the myriad of other important uses we have discovered for hemp.

Hemp is an extremely versatile plant. In fact, back in 1938, *Popular Mechanics* magazine touted hemp as "the new billion-dollar crop," stating that it "can be used to produce more than 25,000 products, ranging from dynamite to Cellophane." Here are just a few of the most exciting applications for hemp:

- Hempcrete (insulation for construction)

- Plastic

- Clothing (antibacterial and odor fighting)

- Energy storage as a superconductor

- Biofuel

- Food (seeds, oil, protein)

Hemp vs. Cannabis: The Entourage Effect

This is where the debate on hemp versus cannabis CBD really heats up, because the main argument boils down to the entourage effect.

A common argument on the pro-hemp side is that "CBD is CBD." The body doesn't care where the CBD molecule comes from, and the molecule is the same whether it comes from hemp or cannabis. This is true, and you can absolutely reap health benefits from the CBD in hemp! But as Samantha Miller, president and chief scientist of the cannabis testing lab Pure Analytics, so eloquently put it: "CBD is CBD is CBD, but the difference is everything else." Meaning, what else is co-extracted from hemp versus cannabis?

The idea behind the entourage effect is that the phyto-chemicals (cannabinoids and terpenes in particular) in cannabis and hemp work better together. They have a synergistic relationship where they help one another and work together to provide a more robust therapeutic effect or health benefit than any one of them could do on their own.

And in addition to that, the proportions of these phytochemicals in any particular strain or even an individual plant will determine a unique therapeutic effect; this is why you'll hear that certain strains are better for sleep or stimulating appetite, while others are prized for pain relief or stimulating creativity. Both hemp and cannabis products can be full-spectrum, meaning they contain CBD and THC in addition to the many other natural phytochemicals present in the plant. Where hemp and cannabis products differ is in the ratios: how much of each of the cannabinoids and other phytochemicals they contain.

Hemp-derived extracts, by law, contain minimal amounts of THC (less than 0.3% by dry weight). While they may also contain measurable amounts of other cannabinoids and terpenes, patient experience is pointing to cannabis extracts as being therapeutically superior, meaning the entourage effect might not be as relevant to hemp extracts.

So the main thrust of the entourage effect argument on the cannabis side is that the phytochemical profiles in

HEALING with CBD

cannabis are richer and more robust, and that the interplay or synergy between compounds like cannabinoids, terpenes, and flavonoids is what provides the highest level of benefit to human health and healing. Hemp can't measure up to cannabis when it comes to the natural presence of these important active compounds.

At this nascent time of CBD science, when patients are really the pioneers of cannabis science and experimentation, the tide of anecdotal evidence seems to be moving toward whole-plant cannabis extracts.

Hemp vs. Cannabis: Growing and Manufacturing Issues

For both cannabis and hemp-derived CBD products, purity and quality come down to the individual farmers and manufacturers, and practices vary widely.

There are both hemp and cannabis farmers working hard to grow clean, organic plants that are safe for human consumption, yet conversely, there are hemp and cannabis farmers who are using questionable practices. Likewise, there are product manufacturers who are taking great care to extract CBD from either cannabis or hemp in ways that are mindful of what residual toxins from the extraction process might make it into their extracts and final products. And there are those who are not so mindful.

According to Martin Lee of Project CBD, CBD oil is actually a co-product or by-product of growing industrial hemp and a way that farmers can make additional money by selling unused hemp biomass:

"This dual-use practice is widespread among large-scale hemp growers in Canada, for example, but it's technically illegal, entirely unregulated, and the hemp biomass sold via underground channels is often tainted with pesticides and requires toxic solvents to extract the CBD."

When much of our source material for making hemp-CBD products comes from abroad, this is a scary thought. Touching upon Lee's mention of extraction methods, this is another area of concern when it comes to cannabis- and hemp-derived CBD. Not all extraction methods are created equally and some of them can be unsafe for consumers (see Chapter 11: Finding Products You Can Trust for an overview on extraction methods).

Another argument that is often made against hemp-derived CBD is in the fact that the plant is a bioremediatory. This means that hemp takes in substances from the soil, both good and bad, through its roots. Like other plants, both hemp and cannabis take in nutrients and water from the soil as well as other contaminants from their environment, including bacteria, fungi, pesticides, and heavy metals. These toxins can remain in the plant if there is too much for the plant to digest, a process called **bioaccumulation**.

The plants hold these toxins in their leaves, stems, stalks, roots, and flowers. When these plants are harvested and processed for consumption, these contaminants can be extremely hazardous to your health, even at low levels. The problem with hemp-based CBD is that the bioaccumulation effect is compounded: It takes a lot of hemp to get a little bit of CBD. This means that, all things being equal, there would be comparatively more toxins in a hemp-derived CBD product than a cannabis one. Without uniform regulations for

HEALING with CBD

heavy metal testing, consumers may be consuming products containing cadmium, lead, arsenic, or mercury, all of which pose serious health risks. This is why sourcing clean and responsibly grown organic hemp *and* cannabis products is so important.

Hemp vs. Cannabis: The Legality Issue

Another hot topic in the cannabis versus hemp CBD debate surrounds legality. Many people think that hemp-derived CBD is legal. Period. If you search for "hemp CBD" or "hemp extracts" on Amazon, for example, you'll find many products that are legal to purchase no matter where you are in the country. And in the midst of a hemp-farming revival here in the US, there are many domestic hemp farmers selling their CBD extracts and products online, shipping to all 50 states. But the quality and amounts of CBD in these products can be questionable.

With cannabis-derived CBD, the legality issue is clear: If you live in a state with no medical program and no adult-use legislation, it is straight up illegal. If you live in a state with a medical program, it's legal for you if you are a registered patient. If you live in a state with a medical program and adult-use legislation, you're aces. It's also very clear that transport across state lines, even from one legal state to another, is not permitted.

When it comes to hemp-CBD, everything gets a lot more complicated. Is hemp-derived CBD legal? The answer to that question is a big, fat, confusing "it depends." Ultimately, it depends on where you live, because CBD laws (even for hemp-derived products) vary by state. So when you see the claim "legal in all 50 states," it's not entirely accurate, even if you can go online, purchase it, and have it shipped right to your door.

Here's why.

In 2014, the Farm Bill (also known as the Agricultural Act of 2014) was passed. It was here that a caveat was added to federal law officially differentiating hemp from cannabis. Under section 7606 of the Act, industrial hemp is differentiated from cannabis as long as no part of the plant (including the leaves and flowers) exceeded a THC concentration of "more than 0.3% on a dry weight basis."

Section 7606 also laid out a legal exception for growing industrial hemp in the United States under the auspices of state-approved pilot research programs. Before then, hemp could not be legally cultivated here. All hemp-derived source materials for manufacture, along with many finished products, were imported from abroad. After the Farm Bill passed, American farmers could grow hemp for the first time in decades, so long as individual states legalized industrial hemp farming and opted into the federally sanctioned pilot research programs.

But at the federal level, all cannabinoids, including CBD, are still technically illegal, regardless of source. In 2016, Congress released a statement in the Omnibus Appropriations Act of 2016 (P.L. 114-113) ("the Funding Act"), which reads:

"None of the funds made available by this act or any other act may be used...to prohibit the transportation, processing, sale, or use of industrial hemp that is grown or cultivated in accordance with section 7606 of the

Agricultural Act of 2014, within or outside the State in
which the industrial hemp is grown or cultivated."

This effectively means that hemp producers operating in a state that is compliant with the Farm Bill can ship their products across state lines with confidence that the DEA should not interfere. DEA spokesperson Rusty Payne even went so far as to say:

"It would not be an appropriate use of federal resources
to go after a mother because her child has epileptic
seizures and has found something that can help and has
helped. Are they breaking the law? Yes, they are. Are we
going to break her door down? Absolutely not. And I don't
think she'll be charged by any US attorney."

OK, great! So states working within the confines of the Farm Bill can legally produce and sell their products, and ship them anywhere in the country.

But, again, the legality issue as it's relevant to you, the consumer, depends where you live.

If you live in a state that has its own hemp laws and is operating under the guidelines of the Farm Bill program, you're golden! You can buy products produced in your state, or buy products from producers in other states who are in compliance with the Farm Bill program. If you live in a state with a medical cannabis program (and you are a card-carrying patient) or adult-use laws, CBD is covered and protected under those laws.

If you live in a "CBD-only" state, things get complicated again. In recent years, 17 states have passed CBD-only laws, which legalize the possession and use of CBD products for specific qualifying conditions—but not cannabis-derived products containing higher levels of THC. CBD-only laws often limit the legal possession and use of CBD products to children with epilepsy, and some nerve and muscle afflictions. Most states with CBD-only laws allow possession, but do not allow licensed dispensaries, home cultivation, or any other supply infrastructure. In other words, registered patients can have it and use it but can't legally obtain it. So if you live in a CBD-only state, you need to know the particular laws of your state. Assuming you are in compliance with those laws, you can source hemp-CBD products.

If you live in a state that has no hemp laws, hemp-CBD products are technically illegal. In these states there are laws against cannabis, and with no hemp-specific laws, hemp falls under the bigger cannabis umbrella. At the time of this writing there are only two states—Idaho and South Dakota—where this was the case. In these two states without hemp, CBD-only, or medical/adult-use cannabis laws, CBD remains a drug that's punishable, in theory, by law.

So, to reiterate, if you live in a state with no hemp laws, or in a state with CBD-only laws, you need to understand the laws applicable in your state and make choices for acquiring hemp-CBD that you are personally comfortable with.

As of this writing, new legislation is being fast-tracked through the Senate to legalize hemp farming. The Hemp Farming Act of 2018 was introduced in April and will legally differentiate industrial hemp from cannabis, allowing for its cultivation and commercial use. It would remove non-psychoactive cannabis varieties known as hemp from the Controlled Substances Act, making hemp-derived, CBD-rich extracts legal.

The Act will also establish hemp as an agricultural commodity, protect state regimes, add crop insurance, and bolster research. The bill would allow states to regulate hemp, while also allowing hemp researchers to apply for grants from the Agriculture Department, according to the office of Senate Majority Leader Mitch McConnell (R-Ky.). McConnell, along with Sens. Rand Paul (R-Ky.), Ron Wyden (D-Ore.), and Jeff Merkley (D-Ore.), support the legislation.

"By legalizing hemp and empowering states to conduct their own oversight plans, we can give the hemp industry the tools necessary to create jobs and new opportunities for farmers and manufacturers around the country," McConnell said in a public statement.

CHAPTER 8

CBD and 27 Major Health Conditions

Our understanding of the human body and the advancements in healthcare have produced a population that lives twice as long as it did just 100 hundred years ago. We now have the knowledge and technology to optimize our bodies to their near full potential. Getting a clear understanding of balance, as it relates to your body and its fundamental functions, will help you along this path.

What is balance and why is it important? Your body works tirelessly to maintain homeostasis to keep you happy, healthy, and disease free. The endocannabinoid system is integral to this work, as are other important systems like the endocrine, renal, and lymphatic systems. Internal balance is as integral to your overall health and well-being as external balance is, and as you probably know, the two are interdependent. Now, this isn't meant to be a self-help book, but this concept is essential to grab hold of. Being able to wake up and be present, comfortable, and pain-free within your body will enable you to show up and put your best foot forward each and every day.

The American diet can contain up to 70% highly processed foods. If you are like three-quarters of the US population, you have a bottle of multivitamins sitting in your kitchen cabinet. Because of an inadequate diet or to fight off a bad cold, many of us feel like we need the added boost of vitamins to stay out of the doctor's office and get out the door to work each day. If taken at the right times and with the right foods, supplements are an important step you can take to improve your health. After the generic multivitamin, omega-3/DHA, glucosamine, echinacea, flaxseed oil, and ginseng are among the top dietary supplements in the country.

Are you looking for an improvement in your overall health and wellness? More energy? More mental clarity and focus? Less anxiety? Better sleep? If you have a need, chances are there is a health supplement for that.

Because of the way they are used by our bodies, canna-binoids can do the job of many supplements (and some pharmaceuticals, to boot). It has been my observation over the past decade as a registered nurse that the use of cannabinoids can significantly improve the quality of life of most individuals. When it comes down to it, can we ask for anything more fundamental than that?

So let's turn our attention to one cannabinoid in particular: cannabidiol. The future of CBD is bright! The myriad ways that CBD works its wonders in the body coupled with its nonintoxicating properties make it an extremely valuable therapeutic compound, and as the scientific study of CBD ramps up we are uncovering new and exciting possibilities for CBD all the time. We already know with a good degree of scientific certainty that CBD can be used to treat a number of symptoms and conditions, and we've outlined these for you in the following section.

We've put together a list of the concerns and conditions that have the most science backing them up, but there are several others that show real potential based on preclinical study (see Recent Research: 2016 Onward on page 46). And did you know that CBD can help your furry friends too? It's true; CBD is being used to treat a variety of health issues for pets (see What CBD Can Do for Your Pets on page 156).

Health Concerns and Conditions

This section highlights the health concerns, symptoms, and conditions that currently have the most science backing up the use of cannabis-derived medicines.

We used Uwe Blesching's *The Cannabis Health Index* as a jumping-off point. Blesching is a medical journalist who developed the *The Cannabis Health Index* as an "evidence-based rating system that shows degrees of confidence in cannabis as an effective treatment for a specific condition." Blesching painstakingly collected the credible scientific studies available for each condition, rated each study on its overall quality and credibility, and tabulated the results to create a 5-point rating scale, ranging from possible to actual in terms of efficacy. Blesching looked at cannabis as a whole and did not break it down as far as individual cannabinoids like THC or CBD.

HEALING WITH CBD

From there we cross-referenced his ratings in the *The Cannabis Health Index* with CBD-specific studies to give you information on conditions that have the most evidence to support CBD's use. Many thanks go to the fine folks at Project CBD for their comprehensive list of scientific studies as they relate to CBD and specific conditions.

Addiction

CBD is showing interesting potential in the realm of addiction, and indeed the endocannabinoid system plays a role in drug dependency, particularly as it relates to the modulation of dopamine levels.[29]

CBD specifically has been shown to protect nerve cells from alcohol-induced neurodegeneration, with neurodegeneration being a major consequence of alcoholism.[30] Alcohol-related liver damage has also been shown to be reduced by CBD in animal studies.[31] Another animal study shows that CBD can inhibit the drug-seeking behaviors, anxiety, and impulsivity common in addiction.[32]

Human clinical trials show that CBD can be very effective when it comes to quitting smoking, with the total number of cigarettes smoked per day decreasing by up to 40% when participants were given a CBD inhaler to use when they felt cravings.[33] CBD is also being looked at as a way to alleviate the symptoms of opioid withdrawal,[34] and has been shown to help reduce the nagging memories associated with drug relapse.[35]

On top of all that, considering CBD's general anti-anxiety and neuroprotective properties, its lack of impairment, and its general safety, it shows great promise for treating addiction.

Amyotrophic Lateral Sclerosis (ALS)

Research around CBD and ALS is still in its infancy, though we do know that conventional therapies for ALS work by suppressing oxidative stress and inflammation while providing neuroprotection. CBD offers all these benefits, and it might be useful in prolonging the survival of neuronal cells and preventing progression of the disease.[36] In addition, cannabinoids may help with other ALS symptoms through the promotion of bronchodilation and muscle relaxation as well as improving sleep.[37]

A recent review concluded that the endocannabinoid system seems to be involved in the pathology of ALS.[38] The researchers believe there is great potential for cannabis as a treatment for both the symptoms and the disease itself. In addition, a preclinical study showed that CBD modulates several genes linked to the development of ALS. The same study showed that CBD also modulates the expression of oxidative stress-related genes, and genes linked to ALS-related mitochondrial dysfunction and excitotoxicity.[39]

Asthma

The use of cannabis to treat asthma isn't entirely new, and the bronchodilating abilities of THC have been investigated.[40] CBD is a new area of research, and a recent review of preclinical data suggests that CBD could be useful in treating inflammatory lung diseases by reducing the protein concentration and production of inflammation-inducing cytokines and chemokines.[41] A preclinical study in Brazil supports the use of CBD to modulate the inflammatory response in asthma.[42]

Autism

While anecdotal evidence mounts for the efficacy of cannabis in helping children on the spectrum, science is still lacking. Initial research has shown that alterations in endocannabinoid signaling may contribute to autism,[43] and the CB2 receptor seems to play an important role.[44] An animal study showed that blocking the enzyme that breaks down our own endocannabinoid anandamide improved anti-social behaviors.[45] CBD blocks that same enzyme, meaning it could be helpful. Compelling anecdotal evidence suggests that cannabis can help reduce self-harming behaviors common in children on the spectrum.

Alzheimer's Disease

Evidence is mounting of CBD's efficacy in treating Alzheimer's. The connection between the endocannabinoid system and Alzheimer's has been investigated in several preclinical studies, and in recent years, CBD has been looked at specifically. Its general neuroprotective, antioxidant, and anti-inflammatory benefits make it a natural fit for Alzheimer's and other neurodegenerative diseases.[46]

Preclinical research suggests that CBD can reduce overall damage to the central nervous system and curb the neuroinflammatory response associated with Alzheimer's.[47] CBD has been shown to protect against memory loss and even help restore memory.[48] CBD also promotes neurogenesis.

Research is also looking at how CBD and other phytochemicals can help treat and even reverse symptoms of the dementia associated with Alzheimer's and other neurodegenerative diseases.[49]

This story is from Janet, whose mother was diagnosed with Alzheimer's/dementia in 2016. She worked with Elisabeth Mack, a registered nurse, to treat her mother:

"Mom began to show signs of paranoia, anxiety, fear, and isolation. Her agitation caused doctors to use prescription medications for depression, anxiety, and psychosis. But Mom got worse, lethargic; she was lying in bed instead of walking, talking, and loving others. Our 'sweet Lorraine' was gone.

In November of 2017, Mom got pneumonia and almost died. By January of the next year she was released from skilled nursing with many, many drugs and no ability to talk, walk, or feed herself. Upon return to her facility, no one recognized her; she couldn't smile, was over-medicated, and was a skeleton from weight loss. In February, a miracle happened when a hospice social worker gave me Elisabeth's phone number!

Elisabeth met my Mom right away at her facility. She advised me to start Mom on a 3:1 (THC:CBD) dose two times a day for the first week...After 24 hours, Mom was willing to eat! A few days later her anxiety started to decrease to the point that people at the facility were asking, what's going on? After one week of two doses a day, Elisabeth recommended the bump up to three doses a day. We started right away, and what a difference!

Another week of three doses a day and Mom was actually smiling, eating, and seeming to enjoy her day.

The third week, Elisabeth recommended Mom's dose change to a 1:1 (CBD:THC) tincture three to four times a day and two more times if needed. Well, we are now entering week 3 of the 1:1 tincture (a total of six weeks in treatment). Mom is a different person! She is smiling all the time, hugging whoever will stop long enough to get a hug, feeding herself, and trying to stand up. All her anxiety and fears have faded. She still has the severe memory loss, but even with the decreasing memory, Mom is thinking more clearly and responding better to her environment. The tincture with Elisabeth's careful attention to dosing and encouragement has made 100% improvement in my mother's quality of life! Everyone at the facility asks me, "How can this be?" Mom is also off all but two of her pharmaceuticals, and by the time you hear this story it will be down to one!"

This story is from Eloise Thiesen, an adult gerontology primary care nurse practitioner, who treated Lena for dementia.

"Lena was 89 at the time her daughter approached me. She was diagnosed with advanced-stage dementia and was close to being placed in memory care. Her history included MS, migraines, high blood pressure, and dementia. When I met with Lena's daughter, she informed me that her mother had been on opiates for 40 years and never had adequate pain control. At the time, she was using hydromorphone to control the pain, quetiapine for sleep, and lorazepam for mood. Not only did Lena still complain of pain, she was falling frequently, not

sleeping, and having a difficult time expressing her words. The facility was giving her daughter one last attempt to control her behaviors before requiring her to move to a locked memory care environment.

I met with the daughter and we talked about how cannabis may help her mom. After reviewing her health history, we decided to focus on Lena's pain and sleep. Lena had never used cannabis before. I started her on a low dose of THC and CBD during the day for pain control and a larger dose at night for sleep. Within three months, we had weaned Lena off her opiates and sleep medication. Shortly after, her memory started to return, she stopped slurring her words, she lost 25 pounds, and she no longer complained of pain. Her sleep improved and she was no longer falling down. Lena had such a remarkable response. She continues to do well after three years on cannabis and has maintained the same dosages since she started."

ADD/ADHD

Cannabis medicines to treat ADHD appear to be moderately effective and can help patients focus, though it remains a debated form of medication for young patients.[50]

Studies have shown that ADHD may be caused by an underlying dysfunction of the dopamine transmitter system.[51] There is a profusion of cannabinoid receptors in the areas of the brain associated with attention deficit (the amygdala and hippocampus), and the CB1 receptor seems to be an important therapeutic target. While there is limited data looking at CBD specifically, CBD's anti-anxiety effects could conceivably be helpful to patients, and CBD might also be helpful for treating side effects like nausea that are often caused by prescription drugs.

Anxiety

According to the Anxiety and Depression Association of America, anxiety disorders affect about 18% of the population, and they are the most common form of mental health disorder. Numerous animal studies and mounting patient evidence supports that CBD has powerful anti-anxiety properties. CBD may be beneficial to treat a number of anxiety-related disorders,[52] such as:

- Panic disorder

- Obsessive-compulsive disorder (OCD)

- Social phobia

- Post-traumatic stress disorder (PTSD), see page 147

- Generalized anxiety disorder (GAD)

- Mild to moderate depression, see page 135

As mentioned in Chapter 5: What is Cannabidiol?, CBD works with the 5-HT1A serotonin receptor and acts in a similar way to prescription **serotonin reuptake inhibitors** (also referred to as selective serotonin reuptake inhibitors or **SSRIs**) like Prozac and Zoloft to increase the availability of serotonin in the brain, which can reduce anxiety and boost your mood. In one animal study, Spanish researchers found that CBD may affect serotonin levels in the brain faster than SSRIs.[53]

Another animal study found consistent use of CBD may help the hippocampus regenerate neurons.[54] In fact, research shows that both SSRIs and CBD may promote neurogenesis. This is important, because evidence suggests that severely impaired neurogenesis may influence suicidal behavior. Future research comparing CBD and SSRIs could really open up our understanding of depression and how to treat it.

In one clinical study, Brazilian researchers did a small double-blind study of patients suffering from generalized social anxiety.[55] After consuming CBD, the participants reported a significant decrease in anxiety. Researchers validated the patient reports by doing brain scans, and the scans showed cerebral blood flow patterns consistent with an anti-anxiety effect.

In another small study, researchers had patients suffering from social anxiety disorder perform a simulated public speaking test after a treatment of 300 milligrams of CBD.[56] Participants reported significantly less anxiety, and these findings were supported by anxiety indicators like heart rate and blood pressure. CBD has also been shown to be very effective for stress-related anxiety and anxiety produced by a stressful event.[57]

Researchers have also investigated the role of several common terpenes in cannabis for treating anxiety. Limonene (page 83) is known for its anxiolytic properties by increasing the levels of both dopamine (in the hippocampus) and serotonin (in the prefrontal cortex) via the 5-HT1A receptor.[58] Linalool (page 82) has been shown to have antidepressant and calming effects.[59]

The potent anti-anxiety effects of CBD are also useful for helping with a variety of other conditions and illnesses where anxiety might be a symptom (like PTSD, Parkinson's, fibromyalgia, or multiple sclerosis).

This story is from Eileen, who helped Becky, age 18, navigate treatment for anxiety, depression, and insomnia:

> *"Becky is an 18-year-old female with complaints of anxiety, depression, and insomnia. She had used 10-milligram CBD pills purchased online from a hemp producer when we met. She was educated about medical cannabis, THC, and the various delivery methods available, as well as the medical cannabis program in her state.*
>
> *Becky qualified for medical cannabis card and then had access to not only high CBD pills, vaporized oils and tinctures, but also other varying ratios of THC:CBD medicines.*
>
> *It was recommended that Becky use high CBD medicines to start, along with a trial of a low dose of THC to help with sleep at night. Success was found using just 1 milligram of THC at night an hour before bed, but the CBD tincture taken during the day did nothing for Becky's anxiety or depression. Upon further collaboration, we agreed that vaporized CBD at the initial onset of anxiety might provide the help she needed. The vaporized high CBD oil did help calm Becky's anxiety, often being relieved with just one inhalation.*
>
> *Although cannabis wasn't helpful to Becky's depression, she is currently in therapy and has provided insight and*

education to her current medical practitioners about the benefits and minimal side effects of cannabis medicines."

Arthritis

Over 50 million Americans suffer from arthritis. In fact, arthritis isn't a specific disease, but refers more generally to joint pain or joint disease. There are over 100 different conditions under the "arthritis" umbrella. Osteoarthritis is a very common form of arthritis that begins as mild joint pain and progresses into chronic pain, stiffness, and swelling. It is most common in the aging and elderly. Rheumatoid arthritis, another very common form of arthritis, is considered an autoimmune disease (see also Autoimmune Disease).

A recent review of the large number of preclinical and animal studies confirms CBD's anti-inflammatory effects, and suggests that CBD and THC have synergistic effects for reducing inflammation.[60] A 2014 review of preclinical research shows that the endocannabinoid system is an important therapeutic target for osteoarthritis pain.[61] The fact that cannabinoid receptors are located all over the body, along with the physiological role of the endocannabinoid system in the regulation of pain, inflammation, and even joint function, are the main ways that CBD may help treat arthritis-related pain. A 2016 study using a transdermal CBD gel in arthritic mice confirmed CBD's efficacy for pain relief and reduced inflammation.[62] Another study in mice showed that oral and injected CBD helped prevent the joint damage associated with arthritis.[63]

One small clinical study showed that Sativex, an oral spray containing a 1:1 CBD:THC concentration, was effective in treating pain at rest, active pain, and in aiding with sleep in rheumatoid arthritis.[64]

Autoimmune Disease

Autoimmune diseases refer to hyperactivity in the immune system's response, where antibodies and immune cells attack the body's own tissue by mistake. The cause of autoimmune disease is not known, though it's believed to be a combination of genetic and environmental factors. There are more than 80 different types of autoimmune disease, and they can affect almost any part of the body. Some autoimmune diseases target only one organ; for example, type 1 diabetes damages the pancreas. Other diseases, like lupus, can target one specific area or organ, or can affect several.

The most common autoimmune diseases include:

- Addison's disease

- Celiac disease (Celiac sprue or gluten-sensitive enteropathy)

- Dermatomyositis

- Grave's disease

- Hashimoto's thyroiditis

- Multiple sclerosis

- Myasthenia gravis

- Pernicious anemia

- Reactive arthritis

- Rheumatoid arthritis

- Sjögren's syndrome

- Systemic lupus erythematosus

- Type 1 diabetes

Autoimmune diseases may also have flare-ups, when they get worse, and remissions, when symptoms get better or disappear. Treatment depends on the disease, but in most cases one important goal is to reduce inflammation, making CBD a great therapeutic candidate.

Additionally, CBD has been shown to be effective in treating disorders affecting the overactivation of immune response and its associated oxidative stress.[65] CB1 and CB2 receptors are present in the immune system, though CB2 receptors are more abundant. CBD stimulates these receptors to support regulation of the immune response.

A 2006 review supported research findings that cannabinoids are regulators of the immune system,[66] and additional research suggests that they work to suppress immune response,[67] which is helpful in many autoimmune diseases. Cannabinoids downregulate the production of inflammatory proteins called cytokines.[68] Additional research found that CBD specifically caused levels of pro-inflammatory cytokines to decrease, while levels of anti-inflammatory proteins increased.[69]

Cancer

Cancer can be most broadly defined as a disease in which abnormal cells divide uncontrollably and destroy body tissue.

There are over 100 types of cancer, with the most common in industrialized nations being lung, breast, prostate, and colon/rectal. While cannabis is known for treating symptoms related to cancer and its treatment—like nausea and vomiting, lack of appetite, pain, and insomnia—there is mounting evidence that it can play an adjunctive role in fighting it as well. And by adjunctive, we mean that cannabis and CBD can provide therapeutic benefit or synergistic value to current medical treatment, not that traditional treatments should be replaced with cannabis.

Initial research with CBD shows promising results for various forms of cancer, such as bladder, brain, breast, colon, endocrine, leukemia, lung, and skin cancers. While better quality research is needed (and this can never be overemphasized!), a 2013 evidence review concluded that cannabinoids work to reduce tumor size and interfere with cancer cell migration, adhesion, invasion, and metastasization.[70] CBD specifically has been shown to stop the proliferation of new cancer cells.[71] In a 2012 study, it was shown that CBD can prevent angiogenesis, an important mechanism by which tumors promote the formation of new arteries and veins to provide them with oxygen and nutrients.[72] And a recent study showed that CBD can also increase the efficacy of antitumor drugs.[73]

The synergies between CBD and THC have also been demonstrated,[74] as have the importance of terpenes, flavonoids, and other active compounds in cannabis (see Chapter 4: Cannabinoids and The Entourage Effect for more) for treating cancer. A 2013 study showed that a spectrum of cannabinoids was more effective for treating leukemia, for example.[75]

This story is from Esther, age 49, who was diagnosed with Stage IV breast cancer.

"After researching and learning online about CBD and THC for advanced breast cancer, I reached out to Eileen Konieczny to find out more. Because of her years of knowledge and experience as an oncology nurse and her role as an advocate for CBD/THC, I trust her information.

I went through the process of getting a medical cannabis card and began taking daily doses of two tinctures; one was high in THC and the other was a combination of THC and CBD in a 1:4 ratio. I began this in October 2016, alongside my traditional allopathic treatments, and I am so glad I did! My quality of life is greatly improved with this healing medicine. I feel great!

To date, I seem to tolerate chemotherapy quite well whether or not I'm on these tinctures, but since incorporating them into my routine, I notice many important, positive differences in my constitution: My appetite went from practically nonexistent to actually feeling hunger, desiring food, and enjoying eating reasonably sized portions. I'm maintaining my weight, which helps keep my system stronger and more stable during chemotherapy. The pain from treatments and recovery from procedures has been reduced. I haven't used pain medicine since I started the tinctures.

Nighttime has transformed from disruptive wake-ups to sleeping solidly until my alarm sounds. My body feels centered and aligned, not scattered and out of sync. My energy stays up during the day. I am active and able to accomplish tasks I set out to do without fear of falling apart by early afternoon. My mood is generally elevated because I'm not frustrated by physical symptoms. My oncology caregivers seem surprised that I consistently report feeling so well, considering the harshness and frequency of my treatments. Because of the easeful adjustment of my body to these tinctures, I plan to continue taking them indefinitely. I am curious to see longer term effects through upcoming PET and CT scans versus symptom management."

Concussion, Brain/Spinal Injury

CBD is known to have potent neuroprotective properties, a fact known and even patented by the US government (see page 37 for more information). A 2003 trial used an equal combination of THC and CBD to treat symptoms arising from a variety of different brain and spinal cord injuries, and found it effective in treating pain and muscle spasms, and improving bladder control.[76] In 2012, a study showed that CBD could be useful in the treatment of spinal cord lesions.[77] It has also shown to be useful in treating neonatal brain injury.[78]

Depression

Depression is a mood disorder that is known for its symptoms of persistent sadness, a loss of interest in life, pessimism that can lead to decreased appetite and energy, and suicidal thoughts. Much like the internal mechanisms described in Anxiety (page 127), CBD can help treat depression through its influence on the 5-HT1A serotonin receptors. CBD acts to naturally increase the amount of serotonin available to the body, just like the common serotonin reuptake inhibitors

(SSRIs) that are often prescribed for depression. In 2008, researchers concluded that the endocannabinoid system could provide a novel new way to treat depression,[79] while a 2016 study supported CBD as a fast-acting anti-depressant drug.[80]

Diabetes (Type 1 and Type 2)

Diabetes is a group of metabolic diseases that are known for producing hyperglycemia (high blood sugar levels). There are two main types of diabetes: type 1 and type 2. Both types of diabetes are chronic diseases that affect the way your body regulates blood sugar, or glucose. Glucose is the fuel that feeds your body's cells, but to enter your cells it needs insulin. People with type 1 diabetes don't produce insulin. People with type 2 diabetes don't respond to insulin as well as they should, and later in the disease, they often don't make enough insulin. Both types of diabetes can lead to chronically high blood sugar levels. That increases the risk of diabetes complications.

Over time, high blood sugar levels can cause damage, dysfunction, and even failure of various organs like the eyes, kidneys, nerves, heart, and brain. Diabetic complications that are linked to the endocannabinoid system include blindness, atherosclerosis, kidney failure, heart disease, and neuropathic pain.[81]

Research has shown that CBD and THCV might be useful in stabilizing blood sugars, reducing inflammation in nerves, and reducing the pain associated with neuropathy, though more research is needed.[82] CBD can also decrease the arterial inflammation that is common in diabetes.[83]

In his work with rats, Dr. Raphael Mechoulam and his colleagues also saw CBD not just block the onset of diabetes,[84] but the development of it as well.[85] A 2010 study showed that CBD helped protect the retinas of diabetic animal subjects.[86]

Fibromyalgia

Fibromyalgia is a fairly common and yet largely misunderstood condition affecting the bones and muscles. Its primary symptoms include widespread pain and soreness throughout the body accompanied by fatigue, as well as sleep, memory, and mood issues. While it's not clearly understood, researchers believe that fibromyalgia amplifies painful sensations by affecting the way your brain processes pain signals.

There has not yet been a lot of research looking at cannabis use for treating fibromyalgia. However, because of its potent anti-inflammatory and anti-anxiety properties, CBD might very well be a good option for symptom management and even treatment. There has, however, been some study of the synthetic form of THC for treating fibromyalgia. As of this writing, Canadian institutions had recently carried out two clinical trials looking at Nabilone (synthetic THC) for treating pain, with the results still pending. A review conducted in 2016 showed that Nabilone was not generally well-tolerated by fibromyalgia patients and was not very effective at treating their pain.[87]

A small clinical trial in Israel (26 patients) showed that after about a year of using medical cannabis (not specifically CBD), all of the patients reported vast improvements on all parameters measured, and 50% were able to stop taking prescription medications altogether.[88]

Dr. Ethan Russo hypothesizes that several conditions (fibromyalgia among them) are caused by a general deficiency in our endocannabinoid systems (see Clinical Endocannabinoid Deficiency). He has been at the forefront for investigating cannabis therapeutics and understanding how the ECS fits into the bigger picture of human biology.

There is, however, mounting anecdotal evidence from patients who experience real benefit from cannabis therapeutics in helping manage their symptoms.

Inflammatory Bowel Conditions

Inflammatory diseases like Crohn's, and syndromes like IBS, cause inflammation of the inner lining of the colon. This inflammation can lead to lots of painful symptoms like cramping, bloating, diarrhea, gas, and constipation. Luckily, there is an abundance of cannabinoid receptors, particularly CB2, in the gut. Because CBD interacts with the CB2 receptors, it's got great potential for treating these conditions.

There have been several studies over the last decade or so showing a strong link between the endocannabinoid system and the GI system.[89] A 2016 study showed that CBD might suppress colitis by reducing the activation of T-cells and inflammatory response in the colon.[90] CBD has also been shown to reduce hypermotility (abnormally high activity) in the guts of mice.[91] CBD's ability to interact with other receptors outside the endocannabinoid system (specifically the PPAR-gamma) also makes it a novel candidate for treating inflammatory bowel disease (IBD).[92]

HEALING with CBD

In one 2011 study, colitis was induced in rodents and the results showed that THC was somewhat effective on its own while CBD was not.[93] A lower dose of THC combined with CBD proved most effective, giving more support for the synergistic relationship between the two and the theory of the entourage effect. The combination of THC and CBD also improved colonic muscle movement. Another 2011 animal study showed that administering CBD *after* inflammation was induced reduced the inflammation, while administering it *before* the inflammation was induced prevented it from happening at all.[94]

In fact, many professionals believe there is a strong connection between the ECS and gut. Dr. Ethan Russo believes that deficiencies in the endocannabinoid system can cause a variety of conditions, including IBS.[95]

Migraines

Migraines are recurrent headaches that are moderate to severe in nature, and typically cause pulsating pain that often happens on one side of the head. They can last from hours to days, and are often accompanied by nausea, vomiting, and extreme sensitivity to light and sound. They can be completely debilitating. Migraine sufferers also tend to experience depression, anxiety, and sleep problems. The exact causes are not known, but migraines may be caused by changes in the brainstem and its interactions with the trigeminal nerve, a major pain pathway.

Imbalances in brain chemicals—including serotonin, which helps to regulate pain in your nervous system—may also be involved. Researchers are still studying the role of serotonin in migraines, but serotonin levels in the brain drop during migraines. Migraines may be triggered by a variety of other factors, like hormonal changes, foods, food additives, drinks like coffee and alcohol, stress, and changes in sleep habits.

Recent studies are supporting a link between endocannabinoid system deficiency and migraines.[96] Russo's own work studying the use of cannabinoids for migraine treatment supports this theory.[97] More recently, work done by researchers posits that triggers (mentioned above) initiate a chemical reaction in the brain, one that would normally stimulate the release of endogenous cannabinoids to restore balance. For reasons still unknown, migraine sufferers may not produce endogenous cannabinoids in the face of these triggers. This leads to a cascade of pain-inducing signals within the brain, which causes a dilation of blood vessels and an increase in pressure and swelling.[98]

In a recent study in human patients, results showed that THC and CBD in combination was an effective form of pain relief in high dosages (200 milligrams total).[99] In the second phase of this study, some patients were prescribed 25 milligrams of Amitriptyline, an antidepressant commonly used for migraines, or 200 milligrams of the THC/CBD combination. After three months of use, it was shown that the THC/CBD medicine was most effective in treating acute pain during an attack, as opposed to decreasing the frequency or duration of attacks.

Multiple Sclerosis

Multiple sclerosis (MS) is an inflammatory and autoimmune disease with unclear causes and is characterized by the breakdown of fat-based myelin sheets in the brain and spinal cord, which leads to a degeneration of the nerve fibers. The most commonly associated symptoms of MS are muscle spasms, numbness, weakness, and slurred speech. Acute and chronic pain are also common symptoms.

Over the last decade, we have come to better understand the role of the endocannabinoid system in regulating the neural signaling that controls spasticity, supporting previous research showing that cannabis-based medicines have been very helpful in managing muscle spasms.[100] Cannabis-based medicines have been approved in several states and in 16 countries across the world for treating both pain and spasticity. One of these medicines, Sativex, is a 1:1 CBD:THC plant-based mouth spray developed by GW Pharmaceuticals, and it is currently awaiting FDA approval for use here in the United States.

There isn't a lot of research looking at CBD's specific effects on MS in isolation; however, one study conducted in 2017 with mice showed promising results for CBD's ability to treat and possibly reverse some of MS's degenerative effects in the brain and spine.[101] That said, there have been several studies supporting the use of a THC:CBD combination for spasticity and pain. It seems that the best dosage varies drastically from patient to patient, and that finding the best personal dose for MS symptoms requires some trial and error.

A cross-cultural study looking at American and Israeli MS patients showed that both groups suffered from high levels of stress and experienced difficulty coping with feelings of hopelessness.[102] Later studies revealed that stress seems to be involved in onset, exacerbation, and relapse.[103] Given CBD's effectiveness in treating anxiety (page 127) and depression (page 135), these therapeutic properties could be quite helpful to MS patients.

This is from Diana, age 57, a patient who worked with Eileen to treat multiple sclerosis:

> "I am so grateful to know Eileen! It's because of her my quality of life has changed. A lot of people thought I smoked cannabis. Well, nope; I tried it in high school, never really liked it, and never smoked again. I had heard of people with MS getting great results, but didn't care to go that route, until...
>
> Eileen came to me and explained how today, with all the different types of medical strains, that it could help my MS. At the time, I was not doing well and it was getting worse. I was diagnosed with progressive MS in 1992, and MRIs through the years have shown that the lesions have gone from the left side of my brain to covering my entire brain. I never tried any of the drugs prescribed for MS as I feel they do more harm down the road. At the time we talked, I was struggling so badly. My condition was also creating depression, and I was almost ready to give in to the MS drugs. I felt, at that point, what did I have to lose? She taught me what I needed to know about medical cannabis, the different delivery methods, and about CBD and THC. I have made such positive progress with not only my health but also my quality of life.
>
> I have learned how to figure out what strains work for which ailments and more. I only wish others with MS would realize it's more than one strain or just smoking it. Sure, I have bad days and my pain is way beyond at times. But I know once I figure out which strain to use as

HEALING with CBD

a salve and internally, it will pass. Eileen, you rock and you're an angel. Thank you for believing and sharing this plant's healing power. Thank you for putting yourself out there and fighting for those that need it. I am forever grateful you came into my life six years ago!"

Nausea/Vomiting

There have been many studies showing the efficacy of cannabis in alleviating nausea and vomiting. Many of these studies focus on chemotherapy and HIV/AIDS patients. It is one of the most commonly accepted medical uses of cannabis. The solid science and high success rates in using cannabis for nausea and vomiting led to the development of several synthetically derived versions of THC, most famously the FDA-approved Marinol. These synthetic drugs produce mixed results in patients, which again supports the idea of the entourage effect and that whole-plant natural medicines are more effective than specific cannabinoids on their own.

Less research has been done looking at CBD specifically, though a few animal studies show promising results. Because CBD works indirectly with the serotonin 5-HT1A receptor, preliminary research suggests it can be used to treat nausea and vomiting.[104] Both CBD and CBDA have proven effective in treating both acute and anticipatory nausea, a common form of nausea among chemotherapy patients that currently has no FDA-approved treatment.[105] CBDA can be a thousand times more potent than CBD.[106] CBD also acts as a reuptake inhibitor for our body's own naturally produced cannabinoid anandamide, allowing anandamide to hang around in our systems longer to do its work in restoring homeostasis to reduce nausea and vomiting.[107]

Neuropathy

Neuropathic pain is a particular kind of pain that stems from nerve damage in the peripheral nervous system. This condition is associated with other conditions like diabetes, multiple sclerosis, sciatica, or HIV/AIDS, and can be caused as a side effect of chemotherapy treatments. Neuropathy can create extreme sensitivity to painful stimuli, pins and needles, cold or burning sensations, and numbness, to name a few common symptoms.

A 2015 review suggests that CBD can be effective in treating chemotherapy-induced neuropathy, and that the drug Sativex was effective in treating the neuropathy associated with both HIV/ADS and multiple sclerosis.[119] Sativex is a 1:1 CBD:THC naturally derived pharmaceutical medication available by prescription in several countries.

Obesity

Cannabis can be used as both an appetite stimulant (useful for anorexia or cachexia, which involves weight and muscle loss due to severe chronic illness) and suppressant (useful for obesity). CBD is a general appetite suppressant. It has also been shown to promote the production of healthy "brown fat" (fat tissue packed with blood vessels that help us burn energy and produce heat), and promote lipid metabolism in general, which could be quite valuable in treating obesity.[108]

Parkinson's Disease

Parkinson's disease (PD) is a neurodegenerative disease that primarily affects a person's motor function and movement, and generally affects people over the age of 60. There is no cure for Parkinson's and other related neurodegenerative diseases like ALS and Alzheimer's.

The disease is caused by misfolded proteins in nerve cells, and in the case of Parkinson's, this happens in the part of the brain responsible for movement (unlike Alzheimer's, which affects memory). PD results from the death of dopamine-producing nerve cells in the part of the brain responsible for movement (called the substantia nigra). The ultimate cause of most cases of PD in unknown, though some can be hereditary, and symptoms generally include shaking extremities, loss of balance, stiffness, shuffling steps, and difficulty swallowing, among others.

CBD and cannabis therapies have shown great promise in treating the symptoms of Parkinson's and might also stop or greatly decrease the underlying nerve damage. Long-term daily use of CBD can have therapeutic effects on preventing the onset, halting the progression, and alleviating the symptoms associated with Parkinson's.

A 2014 study of 22 human patients showed a great improvement in symptoms like rigidity, tremors, and slowness of movement, with improvements in sleep and pain reported as well.[109] There is also preliminary evidence that CBD can delay the progression of PD due to its potent neuroprotective, anti-inflammatory, and antioxidant properties. Studies in both 2015 and 2016[110] concluded that CBD can help recover memory deficits induced by brain iron accumulation, which is a feature of several neurological diseases.[111] Another study showed measurable improvement in quality of life and general well-being scores in PD patients after only one week of treatment with CBD.[112]

A meta-analysis conducted by Italian scientists in 2009 concluded that CBD "is a very promising agent with the highest prospect for therapeutic use in treating Parkinson's."[113]

Pain

Of all the many reasons that people seek out CBD today, the most common is pain. CBD is effective for most forms of chronic pain, as well as many forms of acute or short-term pain. Many studies have shown the endocannabinoid system's role in the processing of pain signals.[114]

CBD does not directly stimulate the CB1 receptors that are involved in pain perception (THC does), but it does have potent anti-inflammatory benefits, making it a great candidate for treating many types of pain. It can be used to reduce inflammation at the site of injury (a sprained ankle, for example), or for chronic pain caused by pinched, irritated, or injured nerves (called neuropathy).

One 2008 review assessed how well CBD works to relieve chronic pain. The review looked at studies conducted between the late 1980s and 2007. Based on these reviews, researchers concluded CBD was effective in overall pain management without adverse side effects. They also noted that CBD was beneficial in treating insomnia related to chronic pain.[115] And, as we've outlined in other conditions covered in this chapter, CBD can be useful in treating the pain associated with:

- Arthritis (page 130)

- Multiple sclerosis (page 140)

- Migraines (page 139)

- Diabetes (page 136)

- Fibromyalgia (page 137)

- Inflammation

- Cancer and/or its associated treatments (page 132)

- Parkinson's disease (page 145)

A number of studies show that CBD can effectively decrease the prescribed dose of opioids for pain management, which is terrific news considering that so many people experience negative side effects or develop addictions to these medications.[116] CBD can also lessen the symptoms of withdrawal from opioids.[117]

Anecdotally, many patients report that a combination of THC and CBD proved to be most effective for treating pain, and one study showed that the combination of the two are particularly effective for treating intractable pain (pain that is not responding to traditional medications) from MS and cancer.[118]

Post-Traumatic Stress Disorder (PTSD)

Cannabidiol has been showing very promising results in the treatment of PTSD. While many people label cannabis as a coping mechanism for PTSD patients, the science is saying that it is also an important mechanism for healing.

Not only does CBD have anti-anxiety effects (see page 90) that are very important for patients suffering from PTSD, but research also suggests that CBD might have an important role in storing traumatic memories through the disruption of traumatic memory consolidation in disrupting the way traumatic memories are stored and consolidated.[120] For someone who is suffering from PTSD, these memories often produce symptoms like nightmares, anxiety, flashbacks, and depression. Many PTSD sufferers often present with drug and alcohol disorders, as well (CBD can help with that, too; see Recent Research: 2016 Onward on page 41).

In a 2016 study, CBD injections were found to be effective at reducing "freezing behavior" (a common fear response in prey animals; think deer in the headlights) in rats that had been exposed to strong fear-based conditioning.[121] The rats given CBD were significantly less likely to be fearful when exposed to the same conditions at a later date, suggesting that CBD can be effective at hindering the development of fear around traumatic memories. Evidence also shows reduced levels of circulating endocannabinoids in patients with PTSD. A 2013 study of individuals present at the World Trade Center attacks supports these findings.[122] Increasing the endocannabinoid tone of the body would be helpful for these people.

Another way that cannabis can aid PTSD sufferers is through sleep. Because nightmares are often a symptom of PTSD, a good night's sleep is sometimes impossible. Cannabis and CBD's role as a sleep aid (see Sleep Disorders on page 154) is yet another way it can help with PTSD.

Schizophrenia

There is a growing body of preclinical and anecdotal evidence supporting the antipsychotic potential of CBD, which is great news because the side effects of antipsychotic pharmaceuticals are often severe and unpleasant. It also means that CBD might be useful in treating other psychiatric disorders like bipolar disorder.

Though results are still preliminary and mostly at the preclinical level, research looking at schizophrenia and CBD has been largely positive. In 2015, a systematic review of all CBD and schizophrenia studies concluded:

> *"The first small-scale clinical studies with CBD treatment of patients with psychotic symptoms further confirm the potential of CBD as an effective, safe, and well-tolerated antipsychotic compound, although large randomized clinical trials will be needed before this novel therapy can be introduced into clinical practice."*[123]

A study that looked at CBD and conventional pharmaceutical therapies showed that CBD was an effective antipsychotic, with significantly fewer side effects.[124] As of this writing, there were five recently completed and five active clinical studies, meaning we will be gaining an even clearer picture of CBD's ability to treat schizophrenia soon.

Seizure Disorders

CBD has gained much of its notoriety because of the almost-miraculous results it has produced for many sufferers of epilepsy and other seizure disorders, especially in children. Many children with a seizure disorder have tried several different pharmaceuticals, and varying combinations thereof. The side effects of these drugs can include dependency, over-sedation, and cognitive impairment. In some cases, patients have what is called intractable epilepsy, which means that pharmaceutical drugs just don't work.

This is where CBD has really shone. Charlotte Figi, a young girl with intractable epilepsy featured in Dr. Sanjay Gupta's documentary series *Weed* (2013), brought national attention to the unquestionable benefit CBD can have for seizure disorders. She was also the inspiration for the hemp-based CBD product line called Charlotte's Web.

Cannabidiol as an epileptic treatment has been of interest to researchers since the 1970s. Though studies conducted then and into the '80s aren't generally regarded as scientifically solid, the results in human and animal subjects were promising. Several studies support the idea that endocannabinoid deficiency may play a role in the development of seizures.[125]

According to a recent literature review, since 2013, 10 epilepsy centers in America have conducted research regarding the efficacy of cannabis to treat epilepsy. In most studies, trial doses of CBD were 2 to 5 mg/kg/day. Several such studies have shown that CBD does have efficacy for treatment of epilepsy. Reported adverse effects of CBD were mostly mild, including drowsiness, diarrhea, and decreased appetite. The review also underscored that further research is needed to understand the various mechanisms of CBD's antiepileptic action.[126]

A 2013 study in Colorado of 11 patients found that all of them reported reduced frequency in seizures, with 73% reporting a near-complete, if not complete, reduction.[127] A 2015 survey of 117 parents by pediatric neurologists at the UCLA Medical Center showed that 85% of parents reported a decrease in frequency in their children's seizures, while 14% reported their children were seizure free.[128]

A small clinical study from 2017 enrolled five patients suffering from Sturge-Weber syndrome, a neurological disorder marked by a distinctive port-wine stain on the forehead, scalp, or around the eye.[129] Over the 14 weeks of study, three of five had a greater than 50% reduction in seizures, and three remained on CBD long term after the study was completed. Another literature review conducted in 2017 confirmed CBD's antiepileptic properties and pointed to GW Pharmaceuticals' successful Phase III trials of Epidiolex (a CBD-dominant pharmaceutical-grade liquid cannabis medicine) as "pivotal evidence of clinical efficacy" of CBD.[130] Epidiolex was approved by the FDA in June 2018 and has gained state-level approval in Colorado, though at the time of writing CBD was still being considered for re-classification by the Drug Enforcement Agency (DEA). In order for Epidiolex to be put onto the market and become available to patients, the DEA would need to reclassify CBD from a Schedule I to a Schedule II or III controlled substance (see Chapter 2 for more on cannabis and the Controlled Substance Act).

Because there is a risk of interaction with antiepileptic drugs, patients should consult with their doctors or medical practitioners before beginning treatment with CBD.

This story comes from Janel Ralph, a mother who founded an American hemp company called Palmetto Harmony to treat her daughter Harmony, who suffers from a rare form of intractable seizure disorder:

"Harmony was born in 2007 with a rare genetic condition known as 'smooth brain,' which produces multitudes of seizures that are considered untreatable by modern medicine. I was determined to find a treatment that would improve my child's quality of life. This determination led to the creation of Palmetto Harmony. In 2015, I founded Palmetto Synergistic Research LLC and created a product line aptly named Palmetto Harmony.

I completely altered my life path to become the CEO of an American hemp company that produces full-spectrum high-cannabinoid oils, and a few short years later, both Harmony's siblings and her father also came to work for Palmetto Synergistic Research, making this company a true family-run operation.

Harmony, and hundreds of other children like her, are now able to have a quality of life that never seemed possible in the past. Harmony can go days without any episodes, and her pharmaceutical intake has reduced by 90%. This reduction in pharmaceutical intake has allowed her to become more alert and aware of her surroundings.

With the help of neurological physicians, we have been able to map her brain through quantitative electroencephalographs (QEEGs) and gain evidence that Harmony's brain is now able to function in areas that should not be possible because of her disorder. I will be the first to tell you that this business and these products have saved Harmony's life and have allowed her family to professionally and personally grow closer together. I believe this plant can change this planet for the better as it has changed my family."

Skin Conditions

The skin has a large number of CB1 and CB2 receptors, and in fact, cannabinoid receptors are found in all the different cell types produced by the skin. Not only that, but our naturally produced endogenous cannabinoids, anandamide and 2-AG, are produced in the same concentrations in the skin as in our brains. In our skin, the endocannabinoid system regulates the hair follicles, oil production, sweat glands, and more. For this reason, cannabinoids can be quite useful in the treatment of skin conditions. CBD in particular has shown promise on a number of fronts.

THC and CBD have been shown to reduce skin inflammation,[131] while the endocannabinoid system seems to play a role in allergic inflammation of the skin.[132]

CBD might be useful for acne because it increases the levels of our own anandamide, which in turn reduces the activity of our oil glands. Through different mechanisms, CBD also acts on its own to curb oil glands while providing anti-inflammatory effects.[133] CBD's antibacterial property would be useful for acne sufferers as well. In a 2017 review, it was shown that many of the active ingredients of cannabis could be useful for treating acne, and CBD in particular has great promise as a non-irritating acne treatment.[134]

For psoriasis, CBD seems to stop the overproduction of keratinocyte cells, the skin cells involved in producing the itchy, flaky layers of skin commonly associated with psoriasis.[135]

Sleep Disorders

Poor sleep is, unfortunately, all too common among Americans. Problems with sleeping are among the top medical complaints in the United States, and they are a major health concern. There are 70 different sleep disorders, the most common including:

Insomnia: the inability to fall asleep or stay asleep

Sleep apnea: impaired breathing while sleeping

Restless leg syndrome: tingling, discomfort, and even pain in the legs that increases at night and is relieved by movement

Circadian rhythm disorders: the disturbance of the internal clock and sleep patterns

Parasomnias: abnormal movements and activities while sleeping, including sleep walking and nightmares

Excessive daytime sleepiness: persistent drowsiness during daylight hours from narcolepsy or another medical condition

Poor sleep is also a risk factor for many serious illnesses, and adults who get less than seven hours of sleep in a 24-hour period are more likely to develop chronic health conditions like obesity, heart disease, diabetes, arthritis, stroke, and depression. According to a 2016 study by Dr. Daniel Kripke, prescription sleep medications come along with increased risk for death, cancer, depression, and infection, not to mention the negative side effects associated with them, like excessive drowsiness the next day and dependence.[136]

The role of the ECS in sleep is clear: As the master regulator of our most basic human functions, the ECS has a direct impact on sleep. (Remember, the ECS umbrella includes eat, relax, sleep, forget, protect. See Chapter 3: The Endocannabinoid System for more.) In fact, our own endocannabinoids, anandamide and 2-AG, fluctuate with our natural circadian rhythms. Anandamide levels in the brain are higher at night, where it works with oleamide and adenosine to generate sleep. 2-AG levels in the brain are higher during the day, and it seems to promote wakefulness.

The ability of cannabis to help with sleep has been known and appreciated for hundreds of years, but CBD has impacts on sleep that are only beginning to be understood scientifically. People will often claim that CBD helps them sleep, and yet we've seen scientifically that at low to moderate doses, CBD promotes alertness and wakefulness.[137] So how does CBD help with sleep?

Because CBD has effective anti-anxiety and calming effects, the experience of better sleep with CBD is not because CBD is causing drowsiness, but rather because the anxiety relief and relaxation it provides allows for better quality of rest.

That being said, because of its biphasic properties (see What Does "Biphasic" Mean?, on next page), CBD can have both alerting effects at low to medium doses and more sedating and sleep-producing effects at high doses. Low to moderate doses of CBD that create an alerting effect might be helpful for narcoleptics, or people suffering from excessive sleepiness during the day. In one insomnia study, high doses (160 milligrams) of CBD were shown to improve the length and quality of sleep.[138]

What Does "Biphasic" Mean?

This means that low and high doses of the same substance can have opposite effects. Many cannabinoids have biphasic effects. THC is known for having euphoric effects at lower doses, but can cause anxiety and paranoia at higher doses. CBD can have alerting effects at moderate doses, and sedating effects at high doses. The biphasic effects of cannabinoids underscore the fact that using cannabis therapeutics is an extremely personal process, and finding the right dose for you is part of the process. See Chapter 10: How Much Should I Take for more.

Several terpenes found most potently in cannabis-derived products, and to some extent, in hemp-CBD products, can also work both on their own and with cannabinoids to help promote sleep: terpinolene, linalool, and myrcene all work as sedatives (see Terpenes on page 79 for more information).

What CBD Can Do for Your Pets

In the last few years, pet owners have caught on to the fact that our animal companions can benefit from cannabis therapeutics too. CBD products for pets have become very popular, and many producers of products for us humans have started similar lines marketed for our pets.

But you might be asking yourself, is this all marketing hooey, or can CBD really be useful for my pet?

The answer is, yes! CBD can be useful for your pets, for the same reasons it's useful for you. If you've looked over the science-y chapters in this book, you might remember that all mammals (and many other creatures too) have an endocannabinoid system. There are CB1 and CB2 receptors throughout the bodies of your dogs and cats, ready to make use of the therapeutic benefits of CBD.

The Very Important Differences between You and Your Pet

Size might seem like the obvious answer, and it's absolutely applicable. Your pets are much smaller than an adult human (or even a child) and require much smaller doses than humans do.

Dr. Robert Silver is a licensed and nationally-renowned holistic veterinarian who practiced in Colorado throughout the legalization process for both medical and recreational purposes in that state. On his site, nurseyourpet.com, he lays out general dosing guidelines for pets based on their body weight.

Aside from size, there are also subtle differences between our endocannabinoid systems and those of our furry friends. One is THC sensitivity. Animals are MUCH more sensitive to THC than humans. If they consume too much THC, it can cause toxicity, and while this probably wouldn't be lethal, it can be an extremely unpleasant ordeal for both your pet and you.

How Much CBD Should I Give My Pet?

Your product should be clearly labeled, telling you how many milligrams of CBD is in each bottle or serving (and how much is in each milliliter if you are using a tincture or oil). For oils and tinctures, one dropper equals one milliliter. Start with the low end dose and see how your pet reacts over the next week. If there is a noticeable improvement, you can keep the dose here. If you don't see improvement, or if the improvement at the low-end dose tapers off after some time, move up to the mid-range dose and observe for a week. In Dr. Silver's experience, the low-end dose is usually sufficient, but each pet is different!

Low-End Dose: 0.05mg/pound, twice daily

Mid-Range Dose: 0.125mg/pound, twice daily

High-End Dose: 0.25mg/pound, twice daily

THC sensitivity is especially high in dogs, who have far more cannabinoid receptors in their cerebellum and brainstem than humans and other animals do. These parts of the brain control coordination, heart rate, and respiratory rate (among other things), meaning too much THC can cause seriously unpleasant side effects in dogs. A common sign of toxicity in dogs is something called "static ataxia," which you can identify if your dog seems very rigid and has trouble standing. You should seek medical support if you think your dog has consumed too much THC.

This is why hemp-derived CBD products are favored for pets, because they will naturally have minimal (and as far as your pet's reaction is concerned, negligible) amounts of THC. This isn't to say you cannot give your pet cannabis-derived CBD products containing THC, but you should focus on CBD-dominant products (20:1, for example) and as the old dosage adage goes: start low and go slow. If your pet is suffering from severe pain caused by arthritis or cancer, or if they have cancer-related tumors, more THC might be therapeutically beneficial to them. Consult with a vet if this is the case.

What Can CBD Treat for Pets?

The great news is that CBD can help with many of the same symptoms, conditions, and diseases in your pet as it does for you. CBD's main benefits for your pet are:

- Anti-anxiety

- Anti-inflammation

- Pain relief

- Anti-nausea

- Anti-epileptic

- Anti-cancer

- Neuroprotectant

CBD will be a potent anti-inflammatory that is great for older pets whose mobility has been reduced by stiff and painful joints, or for pets who suffer from inflammatory bowel conditions. CBD is also great for anxious pets because of its wonderful anxiolytic properties. If your pet experiences skin-related allergies or irritations, CBD makes a great all-natural topical option (just make sure they can't lick it all off!).

Because of its anti-nausea effects, a little CBD might be just the thing next time you need to load your pet into the car. Epilepsy is another area where CBD can be helpful for your pets, and it can confer the same benefits for fighting cancer as it does to humans. And on top of all that, it has neuroprotective properties for the brain, which can help your pet's brain (and yours) age more gracefully.

CBD Products for Pets

All you need to do is search "CBD for pets" and a whole whack of options will come up. While there aren't quite as many options as for humans, you can still find a wide range of CBD-infused products for your pet:

- Biscuits, chews, and a whole variety of treats

- Tinctures and oils

- Capsules

- Topical sprays, salves, and butters

Treats are a great way to trick picky pets into eating their CBD, but tinctures and oils will give you the most control over dosing and they can easily be added to your pet's regular food. And of course, topicals are a good option for skin conditions or sore joints.

Sourcing

Just like you must take care in sourcing your own CBD products (see Chapter 11: Finding Products You Can Trust for more), you should make sure that the cannabis or hemp used in CBD products for your pets are grown in clean, organic, and environmentally responsible conditions.

Several companies have been dinged by the FDA for selling CBD-products for pets with little or no actual CBD in them. A list of producers and their infractions is available on the FDA's website, but reputable producers should be able to provide you with certified lab results for their products so you can verify the CBD content.

Another thing to consider when buying treats that have been baked or cooked is that CBD can be evaporated away entirely (the boiling point of CBD is 320–356°F), so ask producers at what temperatures and for how long treats are baked or cooked. Sometimes CBD products will have essential oils added to the mix. Some essential oils have medicinal purposes, so make sure you research any essential oils added to understand why they might be there. Animals can be quite sensitive to essential oil additives, so if you purchase a product with essential oils, monitor your pet's reaction. You should also check labels to see if there are any chemical additives or preservatives in the product.

And lastly, know your extraction methods (see page 202). While CO2 extraction is generally considered the cleanest method, it is also the most expensive. Other methods, when done properly, can provide viable options. When in doubt, ask the producer about their extraction methods and to see their lab testing results (see page 222 for info on how to read lab reports).

CHAPTER 9

Using CBD: Not One Size Fits All

With its huge umbrella of therapeutic benefits, CBD is often referred to as a miracle drug. But as patients, consumers, and producers grow increasingly excited about CBD as a natural medicine, we need to underscore that there is still much to understand and uncover when it comes to CBD, our endocannabinoid system, and how they fit into the complex workings of our bodies. While we are building a better foundation of understanding each and every day, with every scientific study and personal story that is shared with friends and practitioners, we are still refining our understanding of the complex ways that CBD works in specific conditions and situations, and how it interacts with other cannabinoids and phytochemicals in cannabis and hemp.

We also need to recognize the limitations of CBD itself. Yes, CBD can help with or even treat a wide variety of seemingly untreatable symptoms and conditions. This is possible thanks to our endocannabinoid system, the role it plays in the body, and how CBD fits into that bigger picture. CBD works in some pretty phenomenal and impressive ways. But CBD, and cannabis-based medicines in general, are not cure-alls. Cannabidiol can be of tremendous value and bring tremendous healing to many people, but it does have its limitations. Go into the experience with a level head, an open mind, and tempered expectations.

Not only that, but CBD does not work for everyone. The benefits experienced by some can be near miraculous (think Charlotte Figi and many other children with intractable epilepsy) and nonexistent for others. This could be because the product you're using is CBD snake oil (these products do exist, see Chapter 11: Finding Products You Can Trust), you need a different product or dose, or CBD just doesn't work in your body the way you hoped it would.

Using CBD is an extremely personal and individual experience. CBD might work for your anxiety, but it might not for your best friend's; however, it may help her chronic pain. Or, perhaps what's needed is a different dose. Or you may need a cannabis-based medicine rather than a hemp-based medicine (or vice versa!). Or, perhaps capsules will work better for you than a tincture. So you see, CBD's efficacy can vary by person, dose, source, delivery method, and condition. Consequently, each treatment regimen is individual and unique to each person.

CBD is not a one-size-fits-all medicine, and you should treat its use with care, tailoring it to your specific needs and wants. Whether you're taking CBD as an everyday supplement for its general anti-inflammatory and neuroprotective properties, or you're taking it to help control your MS-related spasticity, use it with the respect and consideration it deserves.

Before you begin taking CBD, you should do two things. First, sit down and get clear on why you want to take CBD and what you want to get out of it. This process will help you later on as you work to tailor your treatment regimen. Think about why you're interested in CBD, what you hope to get out of using CBD, and what your priorities are. For example, you're seeking out CBD because you have fibromyalgia, hope to get pain relief and better sleep, and your top priority is being able to function during the day and sleep well at night. These details will help you figure out which products to use, the dosing amounts, and time(s) of day, for starters.

Consider how tolerant you are to the effects of THC. As we've mentioned several times already, THC boosts and complements the efficacy of CBD—they work better together. THC can also be an extremely therapeutic agent for things like fibromyalgia-related pain relief and sleep problems, for example. If you live in a state where you can access medical cannabis and have a qualifying condition, THC could be a valuable component of your CBD-rich medicine and treatment regimen.

That said, in higher quantities, THC's effects aren't ideal for folks who need to work or have clear minds during the day, and in these cases, a low-THC cannabis-derived product (like an 8:1 or a 20:1 CBD:THC tincture, for example) might be just the thing. For some, THC sensitivity is very high and any THC content is a concern. And still others live in states where they can't access cannabis-derived CBD products. In these cases, hemp-derived CBD is an option worth exploring!

Questions to Ask Yourself:

- Why are you seeking out CBD?

- What do you hope to get out of CBD?

- What are your priorities?

- How tolerant are you to the effects of THC?

The second thing you should do is talk to your doctor. If you are currently on any prescription medications, there may come a time when you need to adjust your dose. CBD may boost the availability in your body of the pharmaceuticals you are taking, meaning you might need to lower the dose of the pharmaceutical. It might also mean CBD is not a viable option for you right now.

Be prepared for your doctor to be unacquainted with CBD or medical cannabis in general, so go armed with basic knowledge and evidence—bring this book along to loan to them (Chapters 3, 4, and 5 will be of particular interest)! Or, point them in the direction of the latest studies (PubMed.gov) and ongoing clinical trials (ClinicalTrials.gov). Another option (unless you live in a state with no medical cannabis program) is to find a physician who is acquainted with cannabis therapeutics through your state's medical program. You can see these physicians regardless of whether you want to obtain a medical card. You can also find doctors and healthcare practitioners through the Society of Cannabis Clinicians, the Association of Cannabis Specialists, and the American Cannabis Nurses Association.

Questions to Ask Your Doctor

- What do you know about CBD?

- Will taking CBD affect my current medications? (See page 100 for a list of possible CBD interactions)

- What about if there is THC content too?

And once you start using CBD, understand that it will be a process of trial and error. Like with any medication, you will need to pay careful attention to how it affects you. Because CBD can cause you to feel more awake and alert, avoid taking it in the evening. You might also experiment with taking your dose once per day or splitting it up into two or three doses. You will need to self-titrate (increase your dosage) slowly, all with the aim of getting to your personal "sweet spot," the lowest dose you can manage while achieving full relief and efficacy. Chapter 10: How Much Should I Take? will cover this in more detail.

And finally, you will likely need to experiment with different types of products and brands. As mentioned, you might want to experiment with hemp versus cannabis-derived CBD (if available to you in your state). Or, you might need to experiment with different delivery methods. As mentioned, there are lots of different ways to use CBD, and you can customize how you take it based on personal preferences and efficacy.

A good way to navigate this process is with a journal, so you can record the time(s) you take CBD, how much of which product you took, what delivery method you used, your physical experience, etc.

The biggest takeaway, though, is to relax and enjoy the process. As mentioned, CBD is an all-natural, nontoxic, and safe compound to work with—and it might surprise you! You could find benefits you weren't even seeking out, or it might work better than you ever hoped. And if it doesn't, rest assured knowing that at the very least you are getting the general anti-inflammatory and neuroprotective properties it confers regardless of any other symptoms or conditions you might have. So dig into this next section, and set forth on your CBD journey!

How Can I Take CBD?

The cannabis products landscape has grown in leaps and bounds. As both cultural and legal attitudes toward cannabis and hemp continue to shift, and as cannabis technology continues to move forward, consumers can expect even more abundance of choice for consumption.

Today, people seeking out cannabidiol can enjoy smoking or vaping CBD-rich flower, but they can also gobble down some artisanal dark chocolate, spread some organic salve onto their sore feet, or slip a quick-dissolving strip under their tongues. The variety of ways you can consume CBD are referred to as **delivery methods** by doctors and industry professionals.

These delivery methods (you might also hear them called "routes of administration" in more medical contexts) are categorized by the path (or route) by which CBD is taken into the body: inhalation, ingestion, sublingual absorption, topical absorption, or transdermal absorption. Each delivery method has its own pros and cons, and often people will utilize a variety of methods to optimize the therapeutic effect or better fit into different situations in their daily lives.

Overview of Delivery Methods

	OPTIONS	ONSET (MINUTES)	DURATION (HOURS)	BIOAVAIL-ABILITY
Inhalation	Smoking, vaping	2 to 15	2 to 4	17% to 44%
Ingestion	Edibles, CBD oil, capsules	30 to 90	6 to 8	6% to 15%
Sublingual	Tinctures, strips, tablets, sprays, high-potency oil	15 to 30	2 to 4	6% to 20%
Topical	Creams, oils, salves, balms, sprays	15 to 30	2 to 4	N/A
Transdermal	Patches and gels	15 to 30	4 (gels) 8+ (patches)	~90%

As you're starting, or continuing, your journey with CBD, experiment with different delivery methods and products until you put together the therapeutic puzzle that works for your body and your life.

Bioavailability

Since there are so many ways to take CBD, how do you know which products will work best for you? There are many factors to take into account—why you're taking CBD, the purity and safety of the product, the ingredients, and the potency, to name but a few. There is one factor, though, that many people don't consider when choosing a CBD product: bioavailability.

Bioavailability is a measure of absorption rate: how much of the CBD you've taken actually ends up available for use in the body. It might seem logical that when you take 10 milligrams of CBD, those 10 milligrams end up being used by your body. Unfortunately, this is almost never the case. There are all kinds of variables at play when it comes to absorption rates.

Delivery method is a biggie, because different routes will deliver the CBD to your body in different ways, and some of these ways are just more efficient than others. Different delivery methods allow your body to take in the CBD in different ways and metabolize it to varying degrees before it gets to the bloodstream, and it is through this process that we lose a lot of the compound.

Other factors that will influence the bioavailability of CBD (no matter what the delivery method is) include your own biochemistry and metabolism, what you've eaten that day, the state of your endocannabinoid system, and how frequently you consume CBD or other cannabinoids. As mentioned, all of these factors vary from person to person, day to day, and even dose to dose. The bioavailability percentages mentioned here are averages, and this is a topic folks in cannabis research are still working on to better understand and optimize.

By understanding how different delivery methods work, you can put the pieces of your treatment regimen puzzle together in a way that will not only help you get the most value out of your products but will also work best for your particular needs.

One simple step you can take to up the bioavailability of CBD is through diet. Because cannabinoids are fat-loving (lipophilic) compounds, it has been largely accepted that having healthy levels of saturated fats (long-chain triglycerides) in your system gives cannabinoids higher bioavailability. A few healthy foods rich in these necessary fats include high-fat dairy products, eggs, beef, lamb, pork, avocado, and coconut oil (see page 51 for more information on supporting your ECS with diet). Initial animal study suggests that consuming CBD with some of these fats will significantly increase the bioavailability.[139]

And while bioavailability is a factor worth considering when choosing a product, the most important thing is to select the delivery methods and products that you feel most comfortable with using.

Inhalation

Today inhalation means a lot more than just smoking a joint (and don't worry, we won't tell anyone if you inhale). While you can acquire CBD-dominant strains of cannabis flower and roll them up into a joint if you wish, now you can also vape CBD products.

As a delivery method, inhalation boasts a quick onset of mere minutes and a peak effect in about 30 minutes, which can be quite useful if you're feeling some acute anxiety or are in need of fast pain relief. When you inhale CBD, it goes directly from your permeable lungs into the bloodstream. This makes inhalation one of the best delivery methods in terms of bioavailability, clocking in at upwards of 35%, second only to transdermal products (see page 183).

The downsides for inhalation come from the noxious and carcinogenic substances in the smoke, which also cause irritation the lungs. Smoking is the least healthy option for inhalation; vaping is a better option in this regard. The duration of the therapeutic effects are among the lowest of delivery methods, lasting anywhere from two to four hours depending on how much you consume.

Smoking

Smoking remains the most popular way of consuming cannabis, and with the rise in popularity of CBD, cultivators have been busy growing and cross-breeding strains that are high in CBD. If you live in a state with a medical and/or adult-use program, chances are good that you can find one of these CBD strains at your local dispensary (note: not all medical programs allow for the sale of flower). Here are some popular CBD-rich strains of cannabis:

- Harlequin (5:2 CBD:THC)

- Ringo's Gift (24:1 CBD:THC)

- Sweet and Sour Widow (1:1 CBD:THC)

- ACDC (20:1 CBD:THC)

- Cannatonic (5:1 CBD:THC)

- Pennywise (1:1 CBD:THC)

- Charlotte's Web (24:1 CBD:THC)

- Dancehall (20:1 CBD:THC)

- Remedy (15:1 CBD:THC)

- Sour Tsunami (1:1 CBD:THC)

- Omrita RX (1:1 CBD:THC)

- Valentine X (25:1 CBD:THC)

And as far as accessing different chemovars (see What Does "Chemovar" Mean? below), flower (bud) will offer the widest selection. You can use flower not just for smoking but also making your own tinctures (page 179) and edibles (page 176) at home. So, if you find a particular strain that really works for you, and can obtain flower in a legal state, you make use of it in a variety of ways.

WHAT DOES "CHEMOVAR" MEAN?

Chemovar is a word you might hear when it comes to cannabis plants/flower. It is becoming the preferred term when talking about different strains of cannabis, ousting the former long-standing common categorization of "sativa" and "indica" among strains. As we continue to better understand chemical profiles of particular strains, the word chemovar more accurately articulates that each strain has its own unique chemical makeup and therapeutic profile. In fact, work is being done to classify cannabis varieties based on their chemovars, or chemical profiles.[140]

Smoking is fairly easy, and aside from a grinder and rolling papers, needs little in the way of specialized equipment. If you wanted to, you could also smoke from pipes or water pipes (bongs or bubblers).

Research supports that cannabis smoke is healthier than cigarette smoke, but smoke is still smoke. Because smoking leads to irritation and inflammation in the lungs, it's not a preferable option for many patients, especially if you are already dealing with a compromised immune system or inflammatory conditions. Additionally, the strong odor of

HEALING WITH CBD

cannabis smoke makes this the least discreet of the delivery methods available.

Vaporizing

Vaporizers work by heating the cannabinoids below the point of combustion, meaning no smoke and almost none of smoke's associated toxins are produced. Instead, you inhale a vapor full of activated cannabinoids, which may (depending on temperature) produce a thick cloud of visible vapor.

There are vaporizers available that work with dry flower, concentrates, or both. They heat the flower or concentrate via either conduction or convection. Conduction puts direct heat on the product, and these models are typically small and discreet (think vape pens), relatively inexpensive, quick, and easy to use. A vaporizer that uses a cartridge filled with concentrate will likely be a conduction vaporizer. Simple conduction models allow you to adjust the temperatures between hot, hotter, and hottest type options, but generally don't allow you to set specific temperatures. Inexpensive models might not regulate temperature accurately or consistently, which can cause a small amount of combustion ("smoldering") to happen.

Convection circulates heated air around the product to vaporize the cannabinoids, and results in a more even dispersion of heat. Convection vaporizers are the preferred method when using flower, as they are much better at preserving terpenes. They are generally more expensive and larger than the conduction vape pens, though there are lots of models out there that are portable. Convection models typically have the ability to adjust the temperature with precision, and newer products, like the Pax 3, offer apps that you can install on your smartphone to set precise temperatures. This is an important feature because the various cannabinoids and terpenes have different boiling points, and with precision temperature control, you can consume these compounds in stages. Convection models are generally less discreet but still offer a quick and easy way to medicate.

What Is a Concentrate/Extract?

"Concentrate" is a blanket term used for any cannabis or hemp product where the cannabinoids have been extracted from plant material (often using a solvent) and concentrated into a potent finished product. These products are also often referred to as "extracts." These are both general terms that can be used to refer to a wide variety of products spanning several different delivery methods. The well-known CBD oil or tincture is a concentrate product, as are vape pen cartridges, along with other more exotic concentrates like shatter, wax, and crumble.

When buying a concentrate or cartridge for vaporizing, make sure it's an all-natural product that doesn't contain flavoring or thinning agents. Propylene glycol and polyethylene glycol are common thinning agents added to vape concentrates (particularly in hemp-derived products) that can be carcinogenic when heated and should be completely avoided. If it's not mentioned on the packaging, inquire about the extraction method for the concentrate (and read Know Your Concentrates and Extraction Methods on page 202 before buying a concentrate). Most states require that all ingredients used in the processing of concentrates are included on the product label.

Ingestion

A good place to start when looking at ingestion as a delivery method is with something called the "first-pass effect." Anything that goes into your stomach will be processed by your liver before it's used by the body. The liver performs what is called a **first-pass metabolism** on cannabinoids before they get into the bloodstream.

When cannabinoids take the scenic route and pass through the liver, they undergo changes that affect both the way your body utilizes them and the effect they will have. This is why edibles containing THC have the reputation for being more potent and psychedelic than other forms of consumption. Not only this, but a significant quantity is destroyed by stomach acid or broken down entirely by digestive enzymes and not used by your body at all. Some producers enhance the bioavailability of ingested cannabinoids by protecting the delicate compounds with a ring of starch-derived sugars called cyclodextrins, which encases the cannabinoids in a protective cage.

This is also why onset of action is much longer, anywhere from 30 to 90+ minutes depending on what you ate that day and your metabolism, among other things. The effects will last much longer, too, anywhere from 6 to 8 hours. But because of the "first-pass effect" caused by metabolization in the liver, the bioavailability of anything you ingest is generally much lower, ranging from 6% to 15%. Depending on a person's own GI tract, absorption can be both slow and inconsistent.

Ingestion is a very easy, convenient, and discreet way to consume CBD, and there are all kinds of products available for ingestion. Because of the long duration of effect, ingestibles make a great option for all-day or all-night effect. And for many commercially made products, self-titration is easy because the dosage information is clearly labeled.

Ingestion is also a great option for anyone suffering from inflammatory bowel conditions like IBD or IBS, since the medicine will be delivered right to where it's needed most.

Edibles

The term "edibles" refers to any infused food or drink. It's a fast-growing commercial category, offering everything from macaroons to muffins, gummies to lollipops, energy bars to chocolate bars, honey, and even hot sauce! Edibles can be made with raw plant matter, infused oils and butters, or an extracted concentrate (as is the case for most commercially produced edibles).

Edibles have a certain notoriety among cannabis enthusiasts, and there are many anecdotal stories of patients and consumers alike consuming too much THC in the form of a tasty treat. The good news is that most commercially produced edibles generally label the quantities of cannabinoids in the entire product, and in a single serving. While intoxication isn't an issue with CBD-only edibles, it's still good to know how much you are consuming (assuming, of course, the labeling is accurate and truthful). If you are experimenting with a combination of THC and CBD in your edibles, make sure you follow the sage advice to "start low and go slow": eat a fraction of a single serving and wait at least 90 minutes to see how it affects you.

You can also make CBD-infused oils and butters at home using cannabis flower, and there are more and more cookbooks out there that can help you do it. These "canna-oils" and "canna-butters" can be easily added to your regular meals. Dosing is a little trickier and less consistent with homemade edibles, but if precise dosing isn't a major concern, making your own infusions is a great way to avoid heavily processed commercially made foods.

Edibles are convenient and discreet, and can be easy to carry with you during the day. If you make them yourself, they can be more economical than many store-bought products as well. Just be sure to keep all edible products out of the reach of children and pets who might mistakenly consume them!

CBD Oil (Tincture)

Most CBD tinctures are in fact just CBD-infused oils, and the names "CBD tincture" and "CBD oil" are often used interchangeably. Strictly speaking, tinctures are generally alcohol based, but you will see CBD oils sold as "tinctures," too. Oil-based CBD tinctures are made by infusing a carrier oil (typically olive oil, coconut oil, medium-chain triglycerides (MCT) oil, or hemp oil) with an extracted concentrate coming from either cannabis or hemp.

While tinctures are generally taken sublingually, CBD oils can also be ingested like an edible or capsule, making oil-based CBD tinctures pretty versatile. In addition to holding it under your tongue or sloshing it around your mouth, you can add your CBD oil tincture to smoothies, yogurt, or even your coffee with cream—anything that you're going to ingest (remember that fatty foods are ideal candidates for upping the bioavailability!).

Capsules. Capsules are another great option for ingesting your daily dose of CBD! Capsules are filled with CBD-infused oil, and they are especially convenient, portable, and discreet with standardized and consistent dosing, to boot. They offer all the benefits of edibles but without the extra calories.

Juicing

Juicing is becoming an increasingly popular way of ingesting cannabis. Cannabis and hemp are technically vegetables, and the raw plants offer many of the same nutrients and health benefits as dark leafy greens like kale and spinach: iron, fiber, calcium, and lots of potent antioxidants.

Not only that, but cannabis juice gives you all the benefits of cannabinoids like CBD and THC, but in their non-active acidic state (see Cannabinoid Acids on page 74 for more). Juicing might be healthiest way to ingest CBDA, offering the most bang for your buck in terms of potency. Unfortunately, juicing requires fresh raw leaves and that makes it most accessible in states where growing your own (clean, organic) cannabis is legal. Check your state's medical and adult-use laws to see if it's possible for you.

Sublingual and Mucosal

This delivery method relies on the mucous membrane under the tongue and in the cheeks to absorb CBD. Capillaries in the connective tissue diffuse the CBD, which then enters the bloodstream. Because this method avoids the stomach and liver, its bioavailability (6% to 20%) is generally higher than ingestion, though not as high as inhalation. It's also a fairly fast-acting solution, with a 15 to 30 minute onset and a 4 to 6 hour duration. As an in-vitro animal study showed, terpenes like pinene, terpineol, and linalool were well-absorbed by tissue in the mouth.[141]

Tinctures are the classic sublingual medications, and in fact, cannabis tinctures were quite common and popular before cannabis first became illegal in 1937 (see Chapter 2: A Brief History of Cannabis). But today, there are several products that have been designed and optimized for sublingual and oral absorption.

Tinctures

Tinctures are easy, effective, and convenient ways to consume CBD. They are also arguably the best delivery method for self-titration because you can adjust on a drop-by-drop or milligram-by-milligram basis if you need to. Tincture bottles range in size, but most are 1-ounce bottles (30 milliliters). They all contain droppers that you squeeze to pull the tincture up, or a cap that a small oral syringe fits into. Either option allows you to squeeze the tincture under your tongue. Good tinctures will have labeled droppers for exact dosing, but a good rule of thumb to know is that the standard dropper size is 1 milliliter and there are about 20 drops in one dropper/milliliter. Labeling should tell you how many total milligrams of CBD are in the bottle, and how many milligrams of CBD are in one dropper/milliliter. General potency for CBD tinctures is 10 to 20 mg/ml but they can be much higher.

Tinctures are discreet and, as long as you screw that cap on nice and tight, portable, too. You can make your own tinctures at home using very high-proof alcohol (like Everclear) or organic vegetable glycerin. The internet abounds with recipes, tips, and pointers. The only downside to tinctures is that the flavor is often strong and bitter, and alcohol-based tinctures can burn the sensitive tissue in the mouth (try mixing it with honey if this happens). Oil- and glycerin-based tinctures can also be mixed into food and drink, in addition to being taken sublingually. If you're looking to make your own, be sure to source organic food-grade vegetable glycerin, as other glycerin products are often made with GMO corn or soy, or with the by-products of industrial processing.

Lozenges

CBD-infused lozenges are another good way to sneak a little extra CBD into your life. They aren't generally very high potency (most lozenges are about 5 milligrams each) but they are very convenient, portable, and discreet. Plus they take full advantage of the absorbent mucous membrane in your mouth.

HIGH-POTENCY CBD PRODUCTS AND OTHER MEDICATIONS

If you are on any prescription medications and you use a high-potency CBD product, like high-potency oils or isolates, let your medical practitioner know. There may be a greater likelihood of drug interaction. See Drug Interactions on page 100 for more information.

High-Potency Oil

These are products you will generally see available in syringes, and they are often referred to as "oral applicators" or "extract applicators." These super-concentrated oils are very thick, viscous, and typically pretty dark in color. They are made for people who need very high doses of CBD or other cannabinoids (for epilepsy, for example), and the dose is typically the size of a grain of rice, making a clearly delineated syringe the ideal way of dispensing. They are typically taken under the tongue like a tincture for optimal absorption, but they can also be ingested or mixed with carrier oils to make your own capsules or edibles.

Quick Dissolve Strips and Tablets

Two fairly new CBD products are quick-dissolve strips (think breath strips) and tablets. Both these products are meant to go under your tongue, and the dosage generally ranges from 5 to 10 milligrams each. They are another easy, convenient, portable, discreet, and standardized way of taking your CBD.

Topical

Topicals are products applied to the skin for localized relief. These products can be anything from balms, salves, lotions, ointments, sprays, or oils.

CBD has been shown to decrease inflammation, muscle tightness, itching, and sunburn when applied topically. Cannabinoids like CBD applied to the skin do not enter the bloodstream or become available to the body as a whole (so the bioavailability is 0). Instead, they are picked up by the many CB2 receptors in the skin, where they are absorbed locally to reduce inflammation and provide pain relief in a specific area. The onset is relatively quick (10 to 15 minutes) and the effects generally last from two to four hours. Even if a topical product contains THC (which is good for pain relief), because it generally doesn't enter the bloodstream, it shouldn't cause impairment.

Endocannabinoids affect the regulation of oil production in the skin, and CBD may prove a novel treatment for acne.[142] Topicals can also be effective for the pain associated with arthritis, especially in the smaller joints of the hands and feet, or in the elbows and knees. CBD can help treat skin conditions like psoriasis or dermatitis, as well. They are a quick source of relief right where you need it, and they are easy to use.

The strength or potency of topical products varies widely, and so will the effectiveness. The therapeutic effect is fairly short lived, but considering the abundance of topicals, they can make a great add-on or bonus feature to your regularly scheduled CBD programming.

What about Suppositories?

There is no real consensus around the effectiveness of rectal suppositories. The rectal route avoids the liver and "first pass" metabolic effects, provided the suppository has excipients (compounds commonly used in pharmaceuticals that aid in the manufacturing process or enhance bioavailability) that allow for proper absorption of the medication. Cannabinoids are fat-loving compounds that do not absorb easily.

Patients report they are getting relief, and one study showed they were effective at reducing colitis (inflammation of the inner lining of the colon) in rats.[143] Commercially available suppositories that utilize hemisuccinated excipients may prove beneficial to some patients. Hemisuccinated excipients help increase absorption by breaking down fat-soluble compounds into water soluble compounds.

Transdermal

Transdermal products are absorbed through the dermis (layers of skin) and into the bloodstream. They provide a quick onset (15 minutes) and relief over a long period of time. Small quantities are delivered slowly and consistently for an average of 4 hours (gels) or 12 hours (patches), though some patches boast a 96-hour delivery window!

Because the cannabinoids in transdermal products do enter the bloodstream, they have a system-wide effect. This makes them useful for conditions that have generalized pain, like fibromyalgia or diabetic neuropathy, or for managing muscle spasms associated with MS, for example. More and more athletes are using CBD patches to help recover from injury. Most anecdotal reports from patients seem to indicate that they do not pack as powerful a punch as some other delivery methods, and that their effects tend to be more subtle.

So far, the transdermal cannabis market has been mostly focused on patches, as opposed to gels. Transdermal patches are adhesive medicated products that deliver specific doses of cannabinoids. Patches can contain THC, CBD, or a combination of both. Some patches contain other cannabinoids like CBN or acids like THCA. Within the last few years, several new companies have entered the market and consumer interest is growing fast.

Currently, patches on the market are applied to a venous area, like the inside wrist or ankle. Some patches can be cut up to administer smaller doses, which makes self-titration pretty simple. You can remove a patch and its effects will dissipate quickly, within half an hour. Patches are very easy to use, just slap them on and off you go, which makes them approachable options for people who don't want to or cannot smoke or ingest.

While most patch products are available in states with medical or adult-use laws, there are a few hemp-derived CBD patches available online.

CHAPTER 10

How Much Should I Take?

Now that you've got a handle on your endocannabinoid system, what CBD is, how it works its magic, plus all the ways you can take CBD, you're probably wondering: how much do I take, anyway?

Get ready for a very unsatisfactory answer: It depends. And it depends on a few key variables.

First, it depends on your very own endocannabinoid system. Each person has their own endocannabinoid tone. But we can't measure those levels with a simple blood test (yet), so finding the right balance for your body will require some careful trial and error.

Another key variable in figuring out your dosage is the reason you are taking CBD. Are you taking it for general health and well-being? Are you taking it for chronic pain relief? Are you trying to treat muscle spasticity associated with MS? Or perhaps general anxiety? Does your child suffer from an intractable form of epilepsy? All of these situations require different dose ranges, and from a clinical standpoint, we are still figuring this out.

How CBD, and all the active compounds in cannabis and hemp, are absorbed, distributed, metabolized, stored, and excreted from the body is an ongoing area of research. **Pharmacokinetics** refers to how our bodies act upon the medicine, while **pharmacodynamics** refers to how the medicine acts on the body, and these are two areas that doctors and researchers are working to better understand. As we will address, it's also a moving target because the state and needs of our endocannabinoid system changes over time.

Remember, CBD (and cannabinoids in general) is not a one-size-fits-all compound. Dosing with cannabis therapeutics of any form is not like dosing with prescription drugs, at least not yet. While we have a little more experience and scientific support for dosing THC, it's still largely a process of trial and error because of the individuality of every body. Cannabinoids deliver very individualized experiences, and as a result, researchers and physicians alike are rethinking the "one size fits all" model of health in favor of a more customized approach.

The good news is, this chapter will offer some very simple, tried-and-true methods for finding the right dose for you. With some thoughtful experimentation, you can go through this process confidently, because working with a safe, all-natural, nontoxic, and non-intoxicating substance like CBD poses little risk. Keeping a detailed log (see page 246) is a great tool to help you along with this journey.

Talking to Your Doctor

Step one should be consulting with your doctor, especially if you have an existing condition or are taking any other medications (see page 100 for information on possible drug interactions and how CBD might affect your prescription meds).

Your doctor may not know about CBD or cannabis medicines in general. But even if you're already pretty sure they don't, it's still important to ask! The more patients ask about using cannabis, the more doctors will be encouraged to learn about the invaluable medicine that has been pushed out of the conversation by decades of stigma, misunderstanding, and misinformation (if you haven't already, check out Chapter 2: A Brief History of Cannabis for more).

A good strategy is to go to your doctor armed with information and resources (maybe even this book!), so you can clearly and confidently explain to them why you are interested in CBD and how you think it can help you. From there they may be willing to work with you, bone up on the information they need (there are medical textbooks dedicated to the subject, see the Resources section on page 247 for more information), and advise you on using CBD.

If they aren't, don't despair! The internet is a great place to start looking for a healthcare practitioner.

The Society of Cannabis Clinicians and the Association of Cannabis Specialists both offer online directories of practitioners. See the Resources section for the web addresses. If your state has a medical cannabis program, you should also be able to find physicians through that.

Dosing Strategies

Figuring out the right individual dose of CBD or any cannabis medicine will be a process, one you need to be actively engaged in and monitor closely to make the most out of these therapeutic compounds. Here are some strategies, tips, and tools to help you do just that!

Start Low and Go Slow

This is tried, tested, and true advice when it comes to consuming cannabis in any form. It's also true for CBD of any form, even with its impeccable safety record and non-impairing properties.

Start low means, not surprisingly, start with a low dose. If you're taking a CBD-dominant product (like a hemp-derived product with negligible THC or a cannabis product with a ratio of 20:1 or higher), this could be as little as 10 milligrams per day to start. If you're using a cannabis-based product with THC and you're a new cannabis consumer, start with a very low dose of THC (1 to 2.5 milligrams), as your sensitivity might be quite high.

When you're starting out, it's a good idea to divide the dose in half, and take that twice daily (perhaps in the morning and afternoon), though some people like to divide the dose and take it three times daily. If CBD creates an alert effect for you, avoid taking it in the late afternoon or evening so it doesn't affect your sleep.

What Are the Ratios All About?

If you're looking at cannabis-derived CBD products, something you are likely to see on product labels are CBD:THC ratios. These express the proportion of CBD to THC, so for example, a 1:1 CBD:THC will be equal parts CBD and THC. If you are looking for CBD-dominant (more CBD than THC) products, you will be looking for CBD ratios higher than 1:1. Common options include 4:1, 8:1, 20:1, and 24:1. While everybody reacts differently, in general the THC effects in a 1:1 may be very noticeable to a novice user where a more experienced cannabis user might find the effect noticeable but not overpowering. A ratio of 8:1 CBD:THC or higher generally provides no impairment. Going up from there, the effects of THC will diminish. The effects in a 24:1 tincture, for example, probably won't be noticeable.

Go slow means give yourself time to assess your body's reaction to a particular dose. Stick with a specific dose for at least a few days and up to a week before upping the amount, and even then, do so incrementally. As you'll find out in the following sections, more doesn't always equal better, and there will likely be a pretty specific range that provides the most benefit to you. Increasing your dose incrementally will make it easier to find that range where you can experience therapeutic effects at the lowest possible dose (you might hear it referred to as the "sweet spot"). The range between the lowest effective beneficial dose and the highest dose where side effects become unpleasant is called your **therapeutic window**.

Deciphering Confusing Product Labels and Dosage Info

With hundreds of products to choose from containing anywhere from one to thousands of milligrams of CBD, the problem of choice might not be your biggest problem! Because there is no standardization or federal requirements for labeling the CBD content of products, deciphering product labels can be very daunting and downright confusing.

Many edible or single-serving products, like the fast-dissolving strips and tablets, will have dosage information by piece or serving size. This makes figuring out the dose pretty straightforward.

Some products, and tinctures in particular, are a whole other ballgame. Without even touching the confusing and misleading way companies are referring/alluding to CBD in their products without calling it CBD (see Chapter 11: Finding Products You Can Trust), the simple math of dosing with tinctures is confusing.

Here are some good benchmarks to know for both dosing AND getting the best bang for your buck:

- Most tincture bottles are 1 ounce (though there are plenty of products that are 2 ounces, 5 ounces, etc.)

- There are 30 milliliters in one ounce.

- The standard dropper size in a tincture bottle is 1 milliliter.

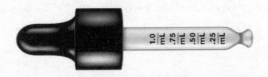

HEALING with CBD

- So, in a 1-ounce (30-milliliter) bottle, there are 30 droppers.

- Each single dropper of 1 milliliter contains, on average, about 20 drops.

With these basic reference points, it's not hard to figure out what you're getting. Many bottles will prominently display the number of milligrams right on the front of the bottle. Let's say the bottle shows 500 milligrams on the front label. This is the total amount of milligrams in the WHOLE bottle. So, if it's a 1-ounce bottle, that means there are 500mg/30ml, or 16.7mg/ml. Since one dropper is one milliliter, that means there are about 17 milligrams of CBD per dropper.

As far as value for your money goes, some products have very low CBD content. Let's take, for example, a 2-ounce bottle of tincture containing 350 milligrams of CBD. While 350 milligrams of CBD might seem impressive, in actuality, in a single dropper you would be getting a maximum of 6 milligrams of CBD (350mg/60ml=5.8mg). Now 6 milligrams of CBD may be just what you're looking for. If not, finding a product with a higher concentration of CBD would be best. Having a higher concentration makes titration easier. In the example above, if you want to double your dosage from 6 to 12 milligrams, you now have to take two full droppers rather than one. With tinctures that are more potent, you can up your dose in fractions of a dropper, or even individual drops.

If you don't see information on the total number of milligrams in the bottle, or the amount per milliliter/dropper, chances are there isn't much CBD in it—if any!

Here are two examples of relatively clear, informative labels:

Supplement Facts
Serving Size 1 ml (1 g)
Serving Per Container: 30

Calories 8.2g	Calories from Fat 8.2 g

Amount Per Serving	% Daily Value*
Total Fat 0.9 g	1%
Saturated Fat 0.1g	0.2%
Monounsaturated Fat 0.1 g	0.2%
Polyunsaturated Fat 0.7g	1%
Omega-6 LA 169 mg	†
Omega-3 ALA 121 mg	†
Omega-9 97 mg	†
Omega-6 GLA 24 mg	†
Omega-3 SDA 12 mg	†
Hemp Oil (Aerial Part Complex) 20 mg	†
Phytocannabinoids 17 mg	†

Not a significant source of saturated fat, trans fat, cholesterol, dietary fiber, vitamin A, vitamin C and iron.

Percentage Daily Value Based on a 2,000 calorie diet
† Daily Value not established

Ingredients: Organic, Cold-Pressed Hemp Seed Ol (non-GMO): Grapeseed Oil: Organic, Cold-Pressed Orange Oi Organic Liquid Stevia (non-GMO): Organic, (non-GMO) Hemp Oil (Aerial Part Complex).
These statements have not been evaluated by the Food and Administration. This product is not intended to diagnose, treat, cure or prevent any disease.

Supplemental information as published on the product Populum Premium Hemp Oil, Signature 500.

Supplement Facts
Serving Size: 0.5 mL
Servings Per Container: 60

	Amount Per Serving	%Daily Value
Calories	5	
Calories from Fat	5	
Total Fat	0.5 g	1%*
Hemp Extract (aerial parts)	43 mg	**

* Percent Daily Values are based on a 2,000 calorie diet.
** Daily Value not established.

Other Ingredients: Fractionated Coconut Oil, Organic Chocolate Mint Flavor Oil (Organic Sunflower Oil, Natural Flavors).
Contains Coconut.

Supplemental information as published on the product Charlotte's Web Hemp Extract Oil, Mint Chocolate 100mL

Because hemp-based CBD is technically considered a supplement, you will see it labeled as such on the nutritional info (as with the label above). You will often see CBD labeled as "hemp extract" in the nutritional info as well, but this isn't accurate—you should ask for and look at the lab results.

Self-Titration, the Biphasic Effect, and Finding Your Sweet Spot

You will often hear the phrase "self-titration" in relation to CBD and cannabis therapeutics, and this is because patients and individuals are working to find their own optimal dosage.

Self-titration means to adjust the dosage of one's own medicine as needed.

As you follow the "start low and go slow" rule we've suggested, you can increase your dosage until you find what people like to call "the sweet spot." The sweet spot refers to the THC dosage where you get the optimal results. Generally speaking, when it comes to any medicine, herbal, or supplement, you don't want to go above the lowest possible dose where you experience the results or relief you are looking for. Why? Well, for one, it will be most cost effective for you. More isn't necessarily better, and higher doses can actually be less therapeutic.

This is because cannabis compounds like CBD and THC are biphasic (see page 156). Opposite effects can be produced with low and high doses, so while a lower dose of CBD might cause you to feel alert, at a higher dose it might relieve your anxiety. Biphasic effects aren't bad; you just need to be aware so you can tailor your treatment plan accordingly.

Experiment with Sources, Delivery Methods, and Ratios

If you've been working with a particular product for a few weeks and still aren't experiencing any noticeable improvement or effect, you might want to try another brand of the same type of product, switch CBD sources (go from hemp to cannabis if you can, or vice versa), or try a totally different delivery method (go from capsule to tincture, or tincture to transdermal patches, for example).

If you're working with a cannabis-derived product, you might want to try a different ratio. As we've discussed, THC has some very potent and wonderful therapeutic effects, especially when it comes to pain relief, muscle spasms, and migraines. The combination of THC and CBD can be an effective one, so if you can tolerate a little more THC it might be beneficial to try. In fact, a recent study showed that adding even a little THC to a CBD-only regimen for epilepsy can significantly reduce the CBD dosage needed.[144]

Start a Journal

A great way to keep track of dosages, different sources of CBD, and different delivery methods is with a journal or log (we've included a sample page for you at the end of this book). Not surprisingly, there are apps for this now, too. Strainprint and Releaf are two such medically focused cannabis tracking apps.

Reevaluate: Hitting a Moving Target

The one thing to keep in mind is that even when you've found your ideal dose, your body, your environment, and as a consequence, your endocannabinoid system and any ailment you might be trying to treat will continue to change. Because of constantly changing variables, maintaining an ideal dosage is often described as trying to hit a moving target. This is why a journal is helpful and why it's important to reevaluate where you're at periodically, so you can adjust as needed.

Tolerance Breaks

If you are using THC as a regular part of your treatment regimen, you might notice the benefits of your medicine diminish over time. This is because our endocannabinoid systems adjust to regular consumption of THC by down-regulating the reception of THC with an overall decrease in the number of CB1 receptors. This reduces its effect on you (see Tolerance on page 194 for more information) and therefore will reduce its therapeutic effectiveness as well, meaning you will either need more medicine or perhaps just not experience the benefits you used to.

Depending on your frequency and quantity of consumption, a few days break might be enough. Research has shown that CB1 receptors start to replenish themselves after just a couple of days, though at least two weeks is considered to be beneficial to really give the body a chance to reset.[145]

If you are treating a severe condition like chronic pain, cancer, or MS, tolerance breaks might not be practical for you, and in fact, building up a tolerance in the face of regular and possibly large doses is beneficial for many patients so they can better manage the impairing effects of THC.

Tolerance breaks aren't mandatory, and building a tolerance isn't necessarily a bad thing. It is just something else to take into consideration when using cannabis therapeutics.

Microdosing for Health and Well-Being

Many folks opt to take low doses of CBD daily as a supplement for preventative care (inflammation is the root of many diseases and ailments, don't forget), general health, and well-being. In fact, many of the recommended dosages on CBD products sold as supplements will fall into the microdose range, between 2 and 5 mg.

While there is no specific science to support CBD as a daily supplement yet, based on what we do know of CBD's universal anti-inflammatory and neuroprotective properties, it makes sense that it would be a good addition to your self-care regimen. We also know that small doses of cannabinoids tend to perturb our CB receptors (rather than binding to them) and stimulate the production of our own endocannabinoids, which in turn creates a more robust endocannabinoid system. Dr. Dustin Sulak, an integrative medicine physician and medical cannabis expert, recommends **microdosing** as a treatment regimen for many of his patients. Microdosing involves the administration of very low doses that are unlikely to produce whole-body effects, but high enough to provide therapeutic benefit. Says Sulak:

> *"Over time, I began to notice that most patients using small amounts of cannabis were getting better and more sustainable results than their high-dosage counterparts with similar conditions. I discovered that most people have a certain threshold dosage of cannabis, below which they'll actually experience a gradual increase in health benefits over time, and above which they'll start building tolerance, experiencing diminishing benefits, and more side effects."*

This is why finding the lowest possible effective dose, or sweet spot, is most easily achieved by the "start low and go slow" approach, and why you might want to experiment with a lower dose as a maintenance dose.

CHAPTER 11

Finding Products You Can Trust

Domestic cannabis and hemp industries still operate in gray areas of the law because regardless of source, all cannabinoids are illegal at the federal level. Cannabis-derived medicines are legal in many states, but at the federal level, they are still very much illegal. This leaves a patchwork of regulatory practices and oversight, with wide variations from state to state, which means wide variations in testing, labeling requirements, product quality, and consumer protection. Hemp-derived products are often touted as "legal in all 50 states," which isn't technically true (see Hemp vs. Cannabis: The Legality Issue on page 113 for more information).

As demand for CBD continues to soar, hemp-derived CBD products are becoming the go-to for patients and consumers who do not have access to cannabis-derived medicines, or who are wary about consuming cannabis. According to *Forbes,* the market is estimated to be worth about $287 million in 2018 and expected to hit $1 billion by 2020. Historically, hemp cultivation has been illegal and has only recently seen a domestic resurgence with new guidelines set out in the 2014 Farm Bill (see page 244). Because of the restrictions and mechanics of the Farm Bill's requirements, American-grown hemp remains a relatively small industry and demand for hemp-derived CBD is at an all-time high.

CBD Products: What to Look For

Whether cannabis or hemp, because the CBD market is new, growing fast, and largely unregulated, there are several issues consumers should be aware of when searching for products. The key areas of concern are:

- Plant-growing conditions. Soil contaminants, heavy metals, pesticides, and molds can all show up in final products.

- Poorly done extractions. These leave behind toxic solvent residuals in final products.

- Inaccurate CBD content labeling. This can take the form of over and under-reporting CBD content, or confusing labeling of CBD content.

- Additives and flavoring agents. This is especially of concern in vape products, where toxic thinning agents are used.

Keep reading for more information on interpreting product labels and lab test results to determine if the product is pure and safe.

To keep up with consumer demand, many of the CBD concentrates used to produce products like tinctures, capsules, and topicals are sourced from hemp grown abroad. In many countries, environmental and consumer safety regulations are less stringent and exporters might not be transparent about their sources or what they contain. Foreign hemp can be residual material leftover from industrial manufacturing, which is often contaminated with pesticides, heavy metals, molds, or microbes. The issue can be compounded by the fact that hemp (and cannabis) plants are bioaccummulators (see page 112), which means that any toxins or contaminants present in the soil will be present in the plant and, when extracted and concentrated, can be passed along to consumers, exposing them to unsafe levels of mercury, lead, and other potentially harmful substances.

In a 2014 statement, the Hemp Industries Association urged American processors of hemp to be cautious:

> *"It is important for American farmers and processors of hemp to understand that most CBD in products mislabeled as "hemp oil" is a co-product of large-scale hemp stalk and fiber processing facilities in Europe where the fiber is the primary material produced at a large scale."*

"God knows what toxins are in the hemp processed in countries like China or Romania, which don't have the same laws about pesticide use that we have," Dr. Ethan Russo told Leafly in 2017. "I don't trust any of it and I don't think anyone else should either."

Because hemp-derived CBD products have flooded the market, the FDA has started evaluating these products, and over the last three years or so has issued warnings to several makers of hemp CBD products for mislabeling, misrepresenting the CBD content in their products, and making unsubstantiated medical claims. In fact, in one sample analysis the FDA did in 2016, only 2 of 24 products analyzed contained the amount of CBD they claimed. While some products only narrowly over-reported the CBD content, some contained no CBD at all.

Another survey of CBD products sold online, conducted by the *Journal of the American Medical Association* in 2017, showed that of 84 different products analyzed, 70% were mislabeled as far as CBD content was concerned. Most of these mislabeled products (42% of the sample of 84) contained more CBD than advertised, while 26% contained less CBD than claimed. Only 30% of the products were accurately labeled. They analyzed vaporizer concentrates, alcohol-based tinctures, and oil-based tinctures. Of these, most of the inaccurate labeling was in vaporizer concentrates where 90% of the products analyzed were mislabeled. The analysis also showed THC present in 18 of the products, and a few had much higher levels of THC than are legally permissible for hemp products (often referred to in the industry as "coming in hot"), which is especially problematic for children or those who undergo work-related drug testing.

Yet another strand in this tangled confusing web is that many producers, including well-recognized and reputable brands, skirt the legality of listing a federally banned substance on their labels. "It's why some manufacturers don't list CBD on the label," says Heather Jackson, CEO and cofounder of Realm of Caring, a patient research and advocacy nonprofit in Colorado. Jackson told Leafly, "They may list 'hemp extract,' which is code for the entire cannabinoid content, but not necessarily CBD."

Because CBD (whether from cannabis or hemp) is still illegal at the federal level, there is no national regulation for product testing, labeling, or safety in the nascent CBD market. Some, but certainly not all, companies volunteer to abide by "current good manufacturing practices" put forth by the FDA. But they are just that, voluntary. Other organizations, like the US Pharmacopeia, consult with all stakeholders to develop guidelines and standards that can be voluntarily taken on by producers, but these voluntary practices are costly for producers to follow and out of reach for many companies. Until there is a more cohesive regulatory framework at the national level, consumers must shoulder the burden of finding clean, quality products themselves. In a landscape crowded with hundreds of CBD products, the majority of consumers don't know what to look for on product labels or ingredients lists, or what information they can ask producers for in order to evaluate the safety of products. It is hard to know who or what to trust.

The product landscape is cluttered with hundreds of brands, options, and delivery methods. There are no reliable dosage guidelines for specific conditions, nor are there standard measurements, which is confusing when attempting to compare products. Adding to the confusion is that most consumers don't have a firm grasp of which delivery system is optimal: Capsule? Tincture? Flower? (See How Can I Take CBD on page 167 for more information.)

In this chapter, we will give you an overview of the key issues currently surrounding CBD products, whether cannabis or hemp derived, as they relate to sourcing, labeling, and ingredients. And we will talk about how you, as a consumer, can obtain the information you need to evaluate products to make sure they are safe for you and your loved ones.

Why Are You Using CBD?

The first thing to consider when setting out to find a CBD product is why you are taking CBD. While more and more people are adding CBD to their everyday supplement routine, there are just as many (or more) who need CBD for more therapeutic purposes—whether for themselves or a loved one they're caring for.

The real issue here is potency. If you are taking CBD as a general supplement or for conditions that need small to moderate doses of CBD, you might prefer lower potency oil-based tinctures, capsules, or edibles. If you are taking CBD for serious conditions like epilepsy, very concentrated products like high-potency oils will be needed and will ultimately be the most cost effective. There are brands and products better suited for therapeutic purposes (full potency, no fillers) and those that make more sense for supplementation, like those with added flavors to improve taste, for example.

Know Your Concentrates and Extraction Methods

Unless you're smoking a CBD-dominant flower, chances are the product you are consuming contains some kind of concentrate or extract. Through extraction, cannabinoids are removed from the plant material and concentrated, which leaves a much more potent substance than the flower itself. The resulting concentrates can be used with much more precision than flower, which makes them ideal for dosing and titrating and can offer patients fast and potent relief.

Depending on the product, it can also be more economical as well.

Depending on the extraction process, other beneficial compounds like terpenes and flavonoids can be extracted along with cannabinoids. The extraction can also be further refined to remove plant materials, chlorophyll, waxes, and other undesirable compounds, or it can be refined to strip away all other compounds to leave a pure CBD isolate. Extraction is a double-edged sword in that the longer and more aggressive the process, the greater the probability both desirable and undesirable compounds may make it into the extract. Though as product markets grow, companies are developing new and innovative techniques for extracting, resulting in more clean and reliable products.

Extraction methods fall into two main buckets: mechanical and chemical. There are many different extraction methods, some so simple you could make them at home (like sifting for kief or using an alcohol solvent for tinctures) and some requiring very expensive specialized equipment along with trained technicians to oversee the process. Each method has its advantages and disadvantages, and knowing your extraction methods will help you make the best decision for your own needs and wants. And regardless of extraction method, if the original plant material was grown using pesticides or in contaminated soil, these toxins will be extracted and concentrated along with everything else— another reason to examine lab results (which you can obtain from any product's producer)!

Let's take a look at the most common extraction methods.

Mechanical Extraction

Mechanical extraction involves physically removing the resinous trichomes (page 105) from the plant and gathering them together to produce a variety of concentrated products like kief, hash, and rosin. Mechanical extraction, unlike chemical extraction, does not use solvents and so you will often hear these referred to as "solventless" or "solvent-free" concentrates. Mechanically extracted concentrates are produced using a variety of techniques, often using sieves, water, heat, and pressure.

Amid the rapidly growing popularity of concentrates and dabbing (consuming highly concentrated extracts) is a strong contingent of consumers who are seeking out solventless concentrates. Because chemical extraction can leave behind trace amounts of the solvent used, some people prefer a more natural product. Kief, dry sieve, hash, and rosin are some of these products.

Kief

Kief is the most simple and easy concentrate to produce. It involves sifting the resinous trichomes through a fine screen that leaves plant material, so in essence kief is just a collection of the resin-filled trichomes. In fact, you can get a three-chamber grinder for home use that will collect kief every time you grind flower, which can then be collected and used on its own. You can also purchase larger screens that the flower can be rubbed into to remove the kief. Kief is a pale powdery substance that can be used to make edibles, or added to smoked flower.

Dry Sieve (Dry Sift)

A more refined version of kief is called dry sieve, or dry sift. It involves even finer screens for filtering and removes the trichome stems, leaving only the round heads where the most clean and concentrated form of the cannabinoid-rich resin is found. It's lighter in color with a fine powdery consistency that can be used in the same ways as kief, and is often pressed into hash.

Both kief and dry sift products can be commercially made with CBD-dominant strains of cannabis and even hemp, though there hasn't been great demand yet for these products. You could, however, produce kief and dry sift at home with CBD-dominant cannabis flower if that is available to you.

Hash (Hashish)

Hash (or hashish) is one of the oldest cannabis concentrates around, produced and consumed for hundreds of years. "Hashish" is also the Arabic word for grass. Though techniques vary, hash is generally made by pressing the mechanically separated trichomes in kief and dry sift. Under pressure, the trichomes burst, and the oily resin inside binds together to form a thick, crumbly, paste-like substance that is most often smoked.

Hash can be made using several different techniques. Ice water extraction is one of the most common processes used to create quality non-solvent hash, and when using this method the most common final product is called "water hash" or "bubble hash." It's made by soaking plant trim or flower buds in ice water and gently agitating the mixture, either manually or mechanically. This forces the trichomes, which become brittle in the icy waters, to fall off. From there they are passed through a fine screen that, like the screens used to make kief and dry sift, filters out most plant matter like ground fan leaves, sugar leaves, and pistils. In recent years, dry ice has also become popular for making hash, and products like the Bubble Bags (or similar competing products) have enabled people to make water hash at home.

Hash is an old school all-natural product that is labor intensive and isn't typically produced at a large commercial scale in North America, having fallen out of favor for more potent concentrates like rosin and other solvent-extracted concentrates like wax, shatter, and honeycomb. It is, however, still a popular form of concentrate in the countries where it has traditionally been used: Afghanistan, Lebanon, Morocco, and India.

Rosin

Rosin is a concentrate that has been gaining popularity in recent years as an all-natural, solventless alternative that retains terpenes and other beneficial compounds from the trichomes. It's made by applying heat and pressure to plant material or kief. With the application of heat and pressure, the resin is exuded from the trichomes and produces a clear amber concentrate. It can be made with either cannabis or hemp, and some domestic hemp growers are beginning to offer hemp-based rosins. As the CBD market matures, we are bound to see more hemp-based rosin products hit the shelves.

Chemical (Solvent) Extraction

The technology and science behind **chemical or solvent-based extractions** has come a long way from the original cannabis alcohol tinctures that graced pharmacy shelves until prohibition in the early 20th century. Today, a variety of solvents are used for these complex "chemical extractions" where they are combined with plant material to strip cannabinoids and other phytochemicals off the plant matter. Depending on how exhaustive the solvent is, other compounds likes terpenes, flavonoids, chlorophyll, and wax can also be extracted from the plant in varying amounts— some methods will extract more, some less. There is no solvent that is ideal for cannabis extraction in every way, and producers will weigh cost, safety, and their desired end results when choosing a method.

As with any extraction method, once the extraction is complete, the solvents are purged from the resinous oil. Purging is a broad term in the world of concentrates, and it can be achieved through evaporation, vacuuming, or hand-whipping. Each method of purging has different variations and produces different end products with varying consistencies. While there are many different options for solvent purging, vacuuming is predominantly considered the most popular. The finished concentrate can be used to produce a variety of products from pure concentrates, from shatter to infusions, CBD oil-based tinctures to edibles. They can also be further refined to remove unwanted plant material like chlorophyll and wax, or to produce distillates and isolates.

Because of varying levels of oversight within the industry, chemical extraction methods have caused concern among consumers in recent years. With the rise in popularity of high-potency concentrates came many poorly made products that often contain remnants of the chemical solvent used— most often butane. However, most reputable producers take painstaking effort to ensure their extracts are clean and well-made. Quality and safety are both influenced by the method of extraction and the skill of the person performing the operation.

As with any product, you can ask the producer for information on their extraction processes, as well as ask to see lab test results, which should list residual solvents (keep reading to find out how to interpret lab tests). Product prices will vary depending on the extraction method, as some extraction methods are more complex than others and require trained technicians and expensive machinery. Supercritical CO_2 extraction is the most costly to producers (and therefore to you) while other concentrates can be produced using relatively inexpensive solvents like ethanol and butane.

Simple Alcohol and Glycerin Extracts

This method dates back hundreds of years: alcohol-based cannabis tinctures were widely used in North America until the early 20th century. Alcohol is a great extraction method because cannabinoids are alcohol soluble. At home, you can make an alcohol-based tincture with a high-proof grain alcohol and decarboxylated (see page 75) ground cannabis flower, but in commercial manufacturing settings the alcohol is often evaporated off to leave behind the concentrated cannabis oil. Alcohol is a safe and easy extraction method, though it is not desirable or appropriate for all patients. In addition, regular sublingual use of alcohol tinctures can irritate the sensitive tissue under the tongue and leave sores.

Glycerin has become a popular alternative for alcohol-free tinctures. Glycerin is a sweet, syrupy substance that is plant derived and chemically related to alcohol, which means cannabinoids can be extracted using it. Be sure the glycerin used is intended for human consumption (it's also used in a variety of industrial processes) and comes from an organic source.

Ethanol

As the name might imply, ethanol extraction also involves alcohol, though you will most often hear about it in the context of commercially produced extracts. The main difference between this and the simple alcohol extraction method described on the previous page is that commercial producers will often purge the ethanol from the oil extraction using specialized equipment.

Ethanol is considered a highly "exhaustive" solvent because it strips cannabinoids, terpenes, flavonoids, chlorophyll, and tannins, among other compounds, from the plant. Chlorophyll is not a desirable compound to extract because it gives concentrates a strong grassy flavor and added bitterness. With further refining, chlorophyll can be removed, but the refining process often lowers the potency of the final product.

Ethanol is more efficient than CO2 and safer to work with than butane, and as a result has become an increasingly popular choice for solvent extraction. The FDA classifies ethanol as "Generally Regarded as Safe," or GRAS, meaning that it is safe for human consumption and commonly used as a food preservative and additive. For reference, the FDA's inhalation limit for ethanol is 16,000 parts per million (ppm).

Supercritical CO2

CO2 extraction is a popular method of extraction among many medium- and large-scale producers and consumers alike because it is a pure chemical substance that occurs naturally and leaves behind no residues. It is widely used by the food, dry cleaning, and herbal supplement industries.

CO2 is nontoxic and is often used as a food additive (in carbonated beverages, for example). CO2 extraction is also used to decaffeinate coffee and tea and extract essential oils for perfumes, among many other uses. The FDA has labeled CO2 safe for industrial extractions, making it a much less controversial solvent than petroleum-based hydrocarbons such as butane or propane.

CO2 extraction offers the most versatility in product development. The solubility of CO2 changes with pressure and temperature, which allows technicians to fraction off different molecules like terpenes and individual cannabinoids. The amounts of these compounds can then be changed and customized. CO2 extraction also provides flexibility in creating an end product, ranging from oils that can be used in edibles, topicals, and vaporizers, to concentrates like wax, crumble, shatter, and sap.

Butane (BHO) and Propane (PHO)

Butane is a common hydrocarbon used for extraction and has been a popular choice among manufacturers because it is relatively inexpensive. Different hydrocarbons (propane, butane, hexane, etc.) have been used since the 1970s for food extractions like corn and canola oil.

Like other solvents, butane is pressurized and run through the plant material to strip the cannabinoids, terpenes, and other compounds. Butane provides an advantage over other solvents like ethanol and CO2 because it is "non-polar," which means that it will not pull out undesirable water-soluble compounds like chlorophyll and plant metabolites. Butane extracts regularly test between 60% to 90% cannabinoid content. The final extract is called "butane hash oil" or "butane honey oil" (BHO).

HEALING with CBD

Propane is rising in popularity and is used in a very similar way to butane. The resulting extract concentrate is called Propane Hash Oil (PHO). Propane offers the benefit of preserving volatile compounds like terpenes. Concentrate end products are similar as well, including wax, budder, shatter, live resin, and more.

Butane extracts have been the main source of concern among consumers in recent years, because of the lack in oversight and regulation that allowed for residual amounts of butane left in the products. Low-quality butane can leave behind an array of toxins that are harmful to humans. When done with proper equipment and oversight, butane extracts are generally considered safe products (see What to Look for in Lab Results).

While butane is generally used for extraction from dry plant material, more recently it has also been used for fresh-frozen plant material, which produces a different extract called "live resin." Live resin is prized for its superior terpene content, flavor, and aroma.

The basic principles of extraction are the same across extraction methods, with the variations in appearance and texture mostly coming from various finishing processes. These finishing processes produce products with different textures, which is where names like honeycomb, shatter, budder, and wax come from.

Products

Once extracted, the resulting concentrate can be made into many different end products. Oil can be infused and used in edibles, vaporizer cartridges, topicals, capsules, and oil-based tinctures, for example. With the rise in popularity of concentrates, extracts are also often used in a dizzying array of other products. While the extracts are generally pretty similar regardless of the extraction method, it is the finishing processes and techniques that create different products. Catching onto the CBD trend, producers are starting to craft CBD concentrates from both hemp and cannabis sources.

Further refinement can produce extracts that can become 99% pure cannabinoid concentrates, called **distillates and isolates**. Distillates typically have a light honey color, whereas isolates tend to be pure white. Isolates are generally available in powder or slab formats, whereas CBD distillates are often packaged in labeled syringes.

When using distillates and isolates you aren't getting the terpenes and other beneficial compounds found in whole-plant extracts, and therefore missing out on all the synergies of the entourage effect (page 77). Distillates and isolates can deliver large doses of medicine in small quantities, which is useful for patients who require them. Some distillate and isolate makers add terpenes back in after refinement for their beneficial effects.

Isolates and distillates can be taken like a tincture, sublingually, or vaporized. They can be added to body oil for topical application (CBD isolate dissolves readily in oil). These products are also odorless and flavorless, which makes them great for adding to oils and incorporated into food and beverages—though avoid heats higher than 350°F, when CBD will boil and evaporate. Honey is a common infusion using CBD isolate powder, but be sure to gently heat the honey in order to dissolve the CBD.

What to Look for on Labels

Products labels are a valuable source of information, even when deciphering them requires you to roll up your detective sleeves and put some work in! Often, what's not on the label can be as informative as what is. The main points of confusion on CBD product labels usually arise from:

- Quantities: How much total CBD is in the product? How much per serving? Is this a good value?

- Source: Where and how was the plant grown? What parts of the plant were used in the extraction?

- Ingredients: What other ingredients are added to the product? Are they safe?

Here we will discuss and provide examples of labels from some of the most commonly used CBD products, such as oil-based tinctures, capsules, and vape cartridges, but these general principles can be applied to any CBD product.

Quantities

For a number of reasons, knowing just how much CBD you are getting in a product can be difficult. With oil-based tinctures, often the total milligrams of CBD will be labeled on the front of the bottle (though you won't often see "CBD" explicitly alongside that number). Sometimes the amount of CBD per serving (usually one dropper) will be provided in the nutrition/supplement facts, and this will tell you how potent the tincture actually is. Potency varies widely among tinctures.

Some quick math to figure out the potency of tinctures if all you have to work with is the total milligram content:

- Tinctures are generally sold by the ounce, and there are 30 milligrams in one ounce.

- Each dropper is approximately 1 milliliter, which means there are 30 droppers in one ounce.

- If your product contains 500 milligrams, then each dropper (1 milliliter) contains 500 mg/30ml = 17 mg.

Other tinctures can be as potent as 50 mg/ml or more. Ultimately it depends on what your needs are, and what your price point is.

The quantity question can be further complicated by the various ways producers label (or don't label) CBD content. While some products are explicit about CBD content by listing it as "CBD" or "cannabidiol" in the nutrition/supplement facts and attaching a number to that, others do not. Some product manufacturers may put "hemp extract," "proprietary blend," or "aerial parts" on the label, and list hemp as an ingredient.

To make matters more confusing, "hemp extract" and "aerial parts" (any parts of the plant exposed to air) don't necessarily reflect CBD content. For some producers it does, but for some it represents total phytocannabinoid content (which would mean there is actually less CBD than listed). This is when having access to lab results or batch results matters because there you will see cannabinoids listed in milligrams per milliliter (mg/ml).

Here are two examples of product labels; the one on the left does not list CBD content, the one on the right does:

Supplement Facts
Serving Size: One Gelcap

One Gelcap Contains:		%DV
Proprietary Blend	1,000 mg	
Hemp extract (seed and stalk) (Cannabis sativa)		*
Clove extract (bud) (Syzygium aeromaticum)		*
Black Pepper extract (fruit) (Piper nigrum)		*
Hops extract (strobile) (Humulus lupulus)		*
Rosemary extract (leaf) (Rosmarinus officinalis)		*

*Daily Value (DV) not established.

Other Ingredients: Gelatin (bovine), Purified Water and Glycerin vegetable source) gelcap.

Supplemental information as published on the product Thorne Hemp Oil +, 30 Gelcaps.

Supplement Facts
Serving Size: 1/2 Dropper
Servings Per Container: 60

	Amount Per Serving	%DV
Full Spectrum Hemp Oil	1 g	*
Cannabidiol (CBD)	10 mg	*

*Daily Value not established.

STORE AWAY FROM DIRECT SUNLIGHT OR HEAT.

Supplemental information as published on the product CBDPure Hemp Oil 600.

With vape cartridges you will probably know the total milligrams of CBD in the product, but not necessarily how much you are getting with each inhale, and this of course varies depending on how long and how many times you inhale. Some producers provide dosage guidelines like this:

Measuring Dosage in 250mg CBD Vape Cartridges							
	2 Second PUFF	3 Second PUFF	4 Second PUFF	5 Second PUFF	6 Second PUFF	7 Second PUFF	8 Second PUFF
Milligrams (mg) CBD per puff*	1 mg CBD	1.5 mg CBD	2 mg CBD	2.5 mg CBD	3 mg CBD	3.5 mg CBD	4 mg CBD
Total puffs in one 0.5ml 250mg cart**	250–260 puffs	170–180 puffs	120–130 puffs	100–110 puffs	80–90 puffs	70–80 puffs	60–70 puffs

*Puffs are measured in seconds counted 1-1000, 2-1000, etc. Milligrams per puff are an approximation and may vary. We cannot and do not guarantee these measurements.
**Total puffs in cartridge are an approximation and will vary. We cannot and do not guarantee these measurements.

Dosage information as published by Green Flower Botanicals for Durban Poison Full Spectrum Hemp Oil Vaporizer Pen Cartridge – 250mg CBD.

One further complicating factor when it comes to quantities is that some companies are mislabeling their products, whether intentionally or not. As mentioned at the beginning of the chapter, consumer watchdogs have been sampling and analyzing CBD products and many product labels misreport the CBD content (and vape products seem to be the most problematic). This is why lab results are a great way to verify that producers are being truthful in their quantity labeling (keep reading to find out what to look for in lab results).

The quantity issue is much easier to navigate with cannabis CBD products because they generally have clear labels that list CBD, THC, and other cannabinoid content.

Sources

Whether from hemp or cannabis, the source of the plant material used to make your CBD product is an important thing to consider.

With cannabis-derived CBD products in adult-use and medical states, the plants will have been grown and products made within the state. From here, you can assess what kinds of growing conditions the plants came from. Today, many products come from organic sources, and this will typically be mentioned on product labeling. Company websites are a good place to look for this information, or you can contact the producers directly to ask about the growing conditions of their plants. Lab results don't lie! As a consumer, you should have access to lab results if you request them.

CBD products bought on the internet that claim they are "legal in all 50 states" are made from either imported hemp or Farm Bill–compliant domestically grown hemp, so the origin of the plant in the product might not be as easy to pinpoint. Often products made using USA-grown hemp will consider this a point of pride and say so on the product label. Products using imported hemp don't generally say so on labels, so producer websites are a good place to go for more information on where their hemp comes from. As we discussed at the start of this chapter, products made using imported industrial hemp can come from large-scale commercial growing operations. These plants can be contaminated with heavy metals, solvents, pesticides, and other toxins—and these contaminants will often find their way into the final product.

Again, it falls on the consumer to do their homework and find out where the plants are from and how they were grown in order to have confidence in what one is using.

Another area of inquiry when it comes to the source of your CBD is what parts of the plant was used in the extraction. In the last section, we discussed product labels that use the phrase "aerial parts." When listed as simply "aerial parts," this could mean that the whole plant (flowers, leaves, and stalks) was used for extraction. You might also see "aerial parts (seeds and stalk)," which is a little more dubious because there is no CBD content in hemp seeds (though they are a good source of polyunsaturated fats, essential fatty acids, and protein!) and there is very, very little CBD in hemp stalks.

CBD BY ANY OTHER NAME

Other names for CBD that you might see on labels: hemp extract, hemp aerial parts, or phytocannabinoids. Be aware that the milligrams associated with these ingredients might not be representative of CBD content.

This could mean the product was made with hemp grown abroad, which may have come from large commercial grows whose end use is for industrial purposes. This could also mean that the hemp was not grown or processed specifically for CBD, but rather CBD is an incidental by-product (and a way to make additional money off a crop). Again, hemp stalk processed for fiber is not meant for human or animal consumption and might have been grown using industrial pesticides and/or in contaminated soil.

WHAT ABOUT "HEMP OIL/HEMP SEED OIL"?

With all the terminology thrown around and used in so many ways by producers, keeping everything straight can make your head spin! Another widely available hemp product is "hemp oil" or "hemp seed oil." This should not be confused with "hemp extract," which is often used on hemp-CBD products. Hemp oil is not a CBD product. Hemp oil is made from the pressed seeds of the hemp plant, which do not contain CBD but are a great source for omega-3 and omega-6 fatty acids. Omega-3 and omega-6 acids also help naturally support your endocannabinoid system (see page 51 for more on diet and your ECS). You can typically tell the difference with size alone; hemp oil is sold in much larger bottles and containers, and is far less expensive than CBD products.

Using the "seeds and stalk" lingo might also be a way for producers to avoid the legal gray area that hemp exists in, since historically any resinous part (flowers and to some extent, leaves) of the hemp and cannabis plants have been deemed illegal. Here are labels from two domestically grown and manufactured hemp products, a tincture (left) and capsules (right). The label on the left calls CBD content "hemp extract" and the one on the right clearly labels CBD content:

Supplement Facts
Serving Size: 0.5 mL
Servings Per Container: 60

	Amount Per Serving	%Daily Value
Calories	5	
Calories from Fat	5	
Total Fat	0.5 g	1%*
Hemp Extract (aerial parts)	43 mg	**

* Percent Daily Values are based on a 2,000 calorie diet.
** Daily Value not established.

Other Ingredients: Fractionated Coconut Oil, Organic Chocolate Mint Flavor Oil (Organic Sunflower Oil, Natural Flavors).
Contains Coconut.

Supplemental information as published on the product Charlotte's Web Hemp Extract Oil, Mint Chocolate 100mL.

SUGGESTED USE:
Take 1 capsule twice daily.

Supplement Facts
Serving Size: 1 Capsule
Servings Per Container: 60

Amount Per Serving	% Daily Value†
CBD (Cannabidiol) 10mg	
Not derived from aerial parts, seeds or isolates.	

† Daily Value not established.

Other Ingredients: Medium Chain Trialycerides (MCT) oil (Coconut and palm), capsule shell
Store in a cool, dark place.

Supplemental information as published on the product Bluegrass Hemp Oil, Genesis Blend – Capsules – 600mg.

Ingredients

Any number of ingredients could be whipped up with CBD, depending on the product. Some products, like tinctures or capsules, tend to be fairly simple, while in others, like edibles, CBD is one of many ingredients. Like all products, some are better than others. The ingredient list is a great place to gather information.

Products like tinctures may have flavors added to make the oil more palatable, and often these are natural essential oils that are known to be safe and used in lots of food products. Some tinctures use artificial flavoring, like bubblegum or cotton candy, to make them more palatable for younger taste buds. Commercially made edibles are processed foods that may have preservatives and other additives, but this varies from product to product. Topicals often have other ingredients added for scent and therapeutic effect. Essential oils like menthol are analgesic and found in many over-the-counter topicals for muscle pain.

Supplement Facts

Serving Size 1 ml (1 g)
Serving Per Container: 30

Calories 8.2g	Calories from Fat 8.2 g

Amount Per Serving	% Daily Value*
Total Fat 0.9 g	1%
Saturated Fat 0.1g	0.2%
Monounsaturated Fat 0.1 g	0.2%
Polyunsaturated Fat 0.7g	1%
Omega-6 LA 169 mg	†
Omega-3 ALA 121 mg	†
Omega-9 97 mg	†
Omega-6 GLA 24 mg	†
Omega-3 SDA 12 mg	†
Hemp Oil (Aerial Part Complex) 20 mg	†
Phytocannabinoids 17 mg	†

Not a significant source of saturated fat, trans fat, cholesterol, dietary fiber, vitamin A, vitamin C and iron.

Percentage Daily Value Based on a 2,000 calorie diet
† Daily Value not established

Ingredients: Organic, Cold-Pressed Hemp Seed Oil (non-GMO): Grapeseed Oil: Organic, Cold-Pressed Orange Oi Organic Liquid Stevia (non-GMO): Organic, (non-GMO) Hemp Oil (Aerial Part Complex).

These statements have not been evaluated by the Food and Administration. This product is not intended to diagnose, treat, cure or prevent any disease.

Supplemental information as published on the product Populum Premium Hemp Oil, Signature 500.

Gives strong, temporary relief from minor arthritis, backache, muscle and joint pain. Helps regain range of motion as pain decreases. Leaves skin soft, smooth and residue free.

Drug Facts

Active Ingredients: Lidocaine 1.65% and Menthol 1.25% (topical pain relief)

Uses: Temporary relief of minor aches and pains.

Warnings: For external use only. Keep out of reach of children. If swallowed get medical help or contact a Poison Control Center immediately.

When using this product: Use on adults or children over age 12. Avoid contact with eyes and mucous membranes, do not use with a heating pad, do not bandage tightly.

Stop use and ask a doctor if: Condition worsens, symptoms last for more than 7 days, or clear up and return within a few days, or redness or irritation occurs.

Other Information: Questions call 1-800-445-6457. Store 20-25C, 68-77F

Directions: Massage into targeting areas of pain and discomfort.

Inactive Ingredients: Water, Canola Oil, Octyl Palmitate, Cannabis Sativa Seed Oil, Sunflower Oil,Emulsifying Wax NF, Fractionated Coconut Oil, Cetyl Alcohol, Dimethicone, Pure Cannabidiol CBD Extract, Anica Extract, Polysorbate 20, Carbomer, Phenoxyethanol, Caprylyl Glycol, Sodium Hydroxide, TEA, IPBC, BHT, EDTA.

Supplemental information as published on the product Biotone 400mg CBD Lab+Blends Pain Relief Maximum Strength Cream 1.76 oz.

An oil-based CBD tincture with natural flavorings (right) and a topical (left)

Vape oils often contain thinning agents like propylene glycol (PG), polyethylene glycol (PEG) or vegetable glycol (VG). There isn't solid research one way or another on the long-term effects of inhaling these compounds. Another consideration is the vaporizer you are using with the oil because not all models have accurate or consistent temperature control, meaning these substances might be "smoldered" at high temperatures, rather than vaporized. We do know that when combusted they can become carcinogenic. Vape oils can also contain flavoring agents, and while these might be safe to ingest we do not know what inhaling these long-term might mean for our lungs.

HEALING with CBD

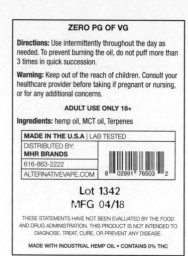

ZERO PG OF VG

Directions: Use intermittently throughout the day as needed. To prevent burning the oil, do not puff more than 3 times in quick succession.

Warning: Keep out of the reach of children. Consult your healthcare provider before taking if pregnant or nursing, or for any additional concerns.

ADULT USE ONLY 18+

Ingredients: hemp oil, MCT oil, Terpenes

MADE IN THE U.S.A	LAB TESTED
DISTRIBUTED BY: **MHR BRANDS**	
616-863-2222	
ALTERNATIVEVAPE.COM	8 02991 76503 2

Lot 1342
MFG 04/18

THESE STATEMENTS HAVE NOT BEEN EVALUATED BY THE FOOD AND DRUG ADMINISTRATION. THIS PRODUCT IS NOT INTENDED TO DIAGNOSE, TREAT, CURE, OR PREVENT ANY DISEASE.

MADE WITH INDUSTRIAL HEMP OIL • CONTAINS 0% THC

Our 300mg CBD Natural Vape Liquid is the highest quality CBD hemp oil in the industry. This new standard is a pure CBD industrial hemp derived oil.

Ingredients: PG, VG, Cannabidiol Concentrate, Natural flavors.

STORE AT ROOM TEMPERATURE, DO NOT REFRIGERATE.

Supplemental information as published on the product American Hemp Oil: 300mg CBD Vape Oil.

Supplemental information as published on the product Alternate Vape: CBD Vape Oil Cartridge 1ml (250mg CBD).

Two vape cartridge labels.

A naturally occurring compound found in cannabis, hemp, and many other plants, terpenes are a popular addition to many vape oils and concentrates. Terpenes are prized for the aroma and flavor they offer, and are a big part of the synergistic relationship that exists between cannabinoids and other compounds in the cannabis and hemp plants. A well-labeled vape oil or concentrate will generally differentiate if added terpenes come from cannabis or hemp (though hemp generally has a much lower terpene profile); from other fruits, vegetables, or plants; or if they were made synthetically.

Terpenes on the plant are present in very small quantities, but we do not know what effects spiking the terpene content of an extract to levels higher than are naturally present on the plant might have on us. At present, there isn't any scientific evidence.

Storing Your CBD Products

CBD is a fragile compound that can be evaporated away if not stored properly. Always keep your CBD products out of direct sunlight in a cool, dark place. Avoid leaving CBD products by windows or in your car. Kitchen cabinets or the refrigerator are good options!

What to Look for in Lab Results

In legal medical and adult-use cannabis markets, third-party testing and analysis is the new standard. Amidst concerns over false labeling of CBD content, plant sources, growing conditions, and possibly harmful additives, the CBD market has been quick to respond.

Permissible Levels and Lab Standards

The permissible levels of potentially harmful substances like heavy metals (which are leeched by hemp and cannabis from the soil), pesticides, fungicides, mold, fungus, bacteria, and residual solvents vary from state to state. Because cannabis (and, until recently, hemp) is a federally illegal substance, state regulators have had no guidance from federal agencies that set health and safety standards for agriculture, food and medicine.

"Some states are regulating it as if it's a pharmaceutical, and some states are regulating it as if it's an agricultural product," Julianne Nassif, director of environmental health for the Association of Public Health Laboratories, a membership organization based in Maryland, told the *Huffington Post* in

2017. This leaves a patchwork of regulation that can look very different from state to state, with some states, like Arizona, not requiring testing at all. Regulators have also had to balance regulations and testing requirements with the cost that fledgling industry and markets can bear.

Pesticide contamination is a common worry for consumers, and yet there is little research on what pesticides can be used with cannabis or hemp cultivation to be used for CBD extraction (as opposed to hemp for industrial uses). When developing regulations, states decide for themselves what can be used on cannabis and hemp plants, setting the maximum allowable levels (also called "action limits") for the list of pesticides they choose.

Most lab tests will also look at microorganisms like fungus and mold. Some organisms, like the fungus *Aspergillus*, have been found on cannabis plants, and this can lead to dangerous infections in people with compromised immune systems. States have generally erred on the side of caution and required testing for the organism. As bioaccumulators, both hemp and cannabis can pull heavy metals from the soil, so you'll see those in lab results as well. Last but not least, you might remember from our discussion of chemical extraction methods, unless purged properly, extracts and any products made from them can leave residual solvents behind.

And, in case this whole story seems too straightforward for you, there are no standards for how the lab testing and analysis itself is actually done. This means that results can vary widely from lab to lab. There are no generally accepted standards for each of the tests, as there are for most other consumer ingestibles and medicines. So producers can favor labs that provide more favorable results. As a result, some states, like Alaska, for example, have found they need to write detailed rules and standards for all laboratories to follow. Sampling can also be an issue, because in some states, growers select and transport samples themselves, which can provide a biased result. Whereas in other states, like Oregon, the laboratories do the sampling, which means more representative and random results.

When looking at lab results, check to see if the lab that produced them is accredited. Reputable labs will be, but not all states require that labs be accredited. Leafly provides an online state-by-state guide of testing standards.

At the industry level, growers and manufacturers feel that regulatory standards should be differentiated to reflect the difference between medical and recreational consumption, whose consumers can withstand different levels of toxins and contaminants.

Lab testing is in an ongoing evolution, and another area where consumers bear the responsibility for doing their homework. If you live in a state with legal cannabis or are buying from a state with a legal hemp program, you should be able to seek out permissible limits from your state department of agriculture.

So to recap, most lab analyses will test for potency, pesticides, microbes, terpenes, residual solvents, and heavy metals.

Potency

This will tell you if the product label is accurate. So if they advertise 1,000 milligrams on the label, are there 1,000 milligrams in the sample tested? Most companies do batch testing, and will include a batch number on the product. Often you will be able to visit their website to track down the lab results for your batch, or you can call and request them. This testing will also show if there are any other cannabinoids present, and in what concentrations.

The lab test results below show the cannabinoid concentrations in a product called Phytocannabinoid Paste 4200 made by Satimed. This product is a highly concentrated hemp-based paste, where 14% of the 30ml (1 oz.) are cannabinoids, for a total of 4200mg. These results show the cannabinoid content broken down by percentages of weight, while you might see other lab tests showing the content in milligrams.

Cannabinoid Potency Values	Test Date	Test Method	Mass, %	Comment
Cannabidiol (CBD)	04/24/2018	HPLC Method	7,22%	Pass
Cannabiodiolic Acid (CBDA)	04/24/2018	HPLC Method	6,56%	Pass
Cannabigerol (CBG)	04/24/2018	HPLC Method	0,14%	
Cannabichromene (CBC)	04/24/2018	HPLC Method	0,49%	
Cannabidivarol	04/24/2018	HPLC Method	0,21%	
Cannabicitran	04/24/2018	HPLC Method	0,35%	
Cannabicyclol	04/24/2018	HPLC Method	0,07%	
Cannabinol (CBN)	04/24/2018	HPLC Method	0,01%	
Total Measured Cannabinoids	04/24/2018	HPLC Method	15,05%	**Pass**

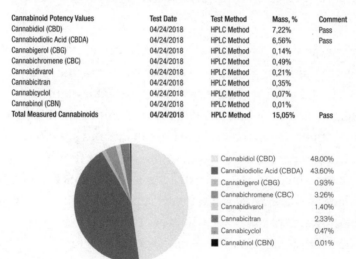

Cannabidiol (CBD)	48.00%
Cannabiodiolic Acid (CBDA)	43.60%
Cannabigerol (CBG)	0.93%
Cannabichromene (CBC)	3.26%
Cannabidivarol	1.40%
Cannabicitran	2.33%
Cannabicyclol	0.47%
Cannabinol (CBN)	0.01%

Lab test results showing the cannabinoid content of Phytocannabinoid Paste 4200 made by Satimed.

Pesticides and Fungicides

This analysis is important for ensuring the safety of hemp and cannabis compounds, as the plants can be treated with herbicides and fungicides, and high concentrations of these substances can be harmful.

These lab results show the pesticide testing. The "nd" under "Mass, %" signifies "not detected," which means that pesticides were present in such low levels they were not detectable or there were none present at all, which is great! While these results do not show the specific list of pesticides tested, many lab results will itemize which pesticides were tested for. Remember that at present, the list of allowable pesticides varies by state.

Pesticides	Test Date	Test Method	Mass, %	Comment
Total Pesticide Residuals by GCh-MS method, mg/kg *	04/27/2018	SDP 5.4.4.Ch.179:2014	nd	Pass
Total Pesticide Residuals by ESCh-MS/MS method, mg/kg **	04/27/2018	SDP 5.4.4.Ch.177:2013	nd	Pass

* - Total 155 Pesticides traces measured
** - Total 153 Pesticides traces measured

Lab test results showing the pesticide content of Phytocannabinoid Paste 4200 made by Satimed.

Microbiological: Fungus, Mold, and Bacteria

Microbiological testing is done to ensure there's no harmful bacteria, fungus, or mold on the hemp or cannabis plants. *Aspergillus, Fusarium,* and *Penicillium* are common molds that are difficult to detect with the human eye and are often caused by poor curing techniques, when the plant flowers are dried for consumption and extraction. *Aspergillus* in particular poses the risk for aflatoxins, a poison produced by some varieties of the mold, which are toxic and carcinogenic. *Aspergillus* can also cause aspergillosis in immunocompromised patients.

These lab tests show the results of "pass" for testing of bacterial content (referred to below as "aerobic microorganisms"), molds, and fungus.

Microbial Test	Date Test	Method	Mass, %	Comment
Aerobic microorganism CFU	04/27/2018	LST EN ISO 4833-1:2013	< 1 x10^1	Pass
Molds and Fungi CFU	04/27/2018	LST ISO 21527-2:2008	< 1 x10^1	Pass

Lab test results showing the fungus, mold, and bacteria content of Phytocannabinoid Paste 4200 made by Satimed.

HEALING WITH CBD

Terpenes

This will provide a detailed breakdown of the terpene profile, the wonderful compounds that give the color and distinctive flavors to the cannabis and (to a lesser extent) hemp plants. Terpenes are pungent oils that provide aromas like cinnamon, berry, citrus, or pine and work synergistically with other compounds in hemp and cannabis to enhance their effects. A terpene profile will look something like this one below, which shows a detailed breakdown of the terpene content, in percentages of weight.

Terpene Profile Values	Test Date	Test Method	Mass, %	Comment
β-caryophyllene	05/17/2018	GC-MS	0,746%	
tetradecanoic acid	05/17/2018	GC-MS	0,406%	
α-humulene	05/17/2018	GC-MS	0,236%	
caryophyllene oxide	05/17/2018	GC-MS	0,235%	
decanoic acid	05/17/2018	GC-MS	0,122%	
cis-β-farnesene	05/17/2018	GC-MS	0,083%	
trans-α-bergamotene	05/17/2018	GC-MS	0,080%	
β-selinene	05/17/2018	GC-MS	0,058%	
n-nonanal	05/17/2018	GC-MS	0,050%	
trans-1,3-dimethyl-cyclohexane	05/17/2018	GC-MS	0,046%	
β-pinene	05/17/2018	GC-MS	0,041%	
α-selinene	05/17/2018	GC-MS	0,037%	
ethyl-cyclohexane	05/17/2018	GC-MS	0,035%	
β-myrcene	05/17/2018	GC-MS	0,027%	
cis-1,2-dimethyl-cyclohexane	05/17/2018	GC-MS	0,024%	
octanoic acid	05/17/2018	GC-MS	0,020%	
allo-aromadendrene	05/17/2018	GC-MS	0,019%	
α-pinene	05/17/2018	GC-MS	0,019%	
nonanoic acid	05/17/2018	GC-MS	0,018%	
β-sesquiphellandrene	05/17/2018	GC-MS	0,018%	
α-zingiberene	05/17/2018	GC-MS	0,016%	
cis-caryophyllene	05/17/2018	GC-MS	0,016%	
dodecanoic acid	05/17/2018	GC-MS	0,014%	
selina-3,7(11)-diene	05/17/2018	GC-MS	0,013%	
2E-heptenal	05/17/2018	GC-MS	0,012%	
para-cymen-8-ol	05/17/2018	GC-MS	0,010%	
trans-nerolidol	05/17/2018	GC-MS	0,010%	
cis-α-bergamotene	05/17/2018	GC-MS	0,008%	
6-methyl-5-hepten-2-one	05/17/2018	GC-MS	0,004%	
terpinolene	05/17/2018	GC-MS	0,004%	

Lab test results showing the terpene profile of Phytocannabinoid Paste 4200 made by Satimed.

Residual Solvents

A complete lab test should also include analyses of the residual solvents. Solvents are used when the plants are processed and turned into oils, powders, or other products, but only for the solvent-based extraction processes. High concentrations of solvents like ethanol, butane, or propane are unsafe.

These results show the residual solvent content, referred to as "Polycyclic Aromatic Hydrocarbons." The types of solvents tested for can vary from state to state.

Polycyclic Aromatic Hydrocarbons by ESCH-FLD method	Test Date	Test Method	Mass, %	Comment
Sum of 4 EU PAH, µg/kg	04/27/2018	SDP 5.4.4.Ch.207:2015	nd	Pass
Benzo-a-anthracene, µg/kg	04/27/2018	SDP 5.4.4.Ch.207:2015 nd	Pass	
Benzo-a-pyrene, µg/kg	04/27/2018	SDP 5.4.4.Ch.207:2015 nd	Pass	
Benzo-b-fluoranthene, µg/kg	04/27/2018	SDP 5.4.4.Ch.207:2015	nd	Pass
Chrysene, µg/kg	04/27/2018	SDP 5.4.4.Ch.207:2015	nd	Pass

Lab test results showing the residual solvent content of Phytocannabinoid Paste 4200 made by Satimed.

Heavy Metals

Heavy metal testing is another way you can determine whether the plants used in your product were grown in safe conditions. Because cannabis and hemp plants are excellent bioremediators, they soak up whatever their roots contact. Even in very small quantities, heavy metals like lead, cadmium, arsenic, and mercury can be harmful to your health.

These test results show that the heavy metals tested for (arsenic, mercury, cadmium, and lead) were not present in detectable levels as shown by the "nd" (not detected) under "Mass, %."

Heavy Metals	Test Date	Test Method	Mass, %	Comment
Total Arsenic, mg/lg	04/27/2018	LST EN 15763:2010	nd	Pass
Total Mercury, mg/kg	04/27/2018	LST EN 15763:2010	nd	Pass
Cadmium (Cd), mg/kg	04/27/2018	LST EN 15763:2010	nd	Pass
Lead (Pb), mg/kg	04/27/2018	LST EN 15763:2010	nd	Pass

Lab test results showing the heavy metal content of Phytocannabinoid Paste 4200 made by Satimed.

Product Pricing

As with any product, prices vary with quality and production cost. Prices for CBD products vary quite a lot, with some companies focusing on producing low-frills, high-quality products, and others investing heavily in unique product formulation, packaging, and marketing. Ounce for ounce, prices for high-quality cannabis or pure CBD are higher than precious metals like gold and many high-end perfumes.

A good way to compare apples to apples is to do some quick math and determine the price per milligram of CBD. Generally speaking, as a consumer you must balance wants and needs with what you are willing to spend and evaluating product safety as part of this process.

Summary: Questions to Ask and Things to Look For

The CBD industry is a booming market, but it is still relatively young. The situation is complicated by prohibition, legal uncertainties, the absence of FDA regulations, and insufficient consumer information. Some companies are producing high-quality, locally sourced, lab-tested, and toxin-free CBD products. Others may be importing cheap hemp oil of unknown quality and slapping a CBD label on a bottle.

With time, stronger regulations will help improve the transparency and quality control behind these products. Low-quality manufacturers will be pushed out of the market, and companies will learn how to increase their quality, decrease their prices, and still turn a profit. But until then, patients and consumers must do their own product vetting.

So to summarize, here are the main takeaways when looking for products:

- Always ask for third-party lab results and look for potency, pesticide, heavy metal, microbiological, and residual solvent testing.

- Pay close attention to product labeling showing the ingredients, quantity of CBD, manufacturing date, and batch number.

- Do your homework and don't hesitate to ask producers for more information.

On the next page you will find an example of full lab test results, with pieces highlighted and explained to put all of this information together.

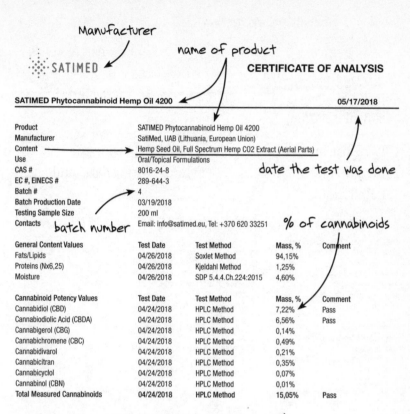

Manufacturer

name of product

∴ SATIMED

CERTIFICATE OF ANALYSIS

SATIMED Phytocannabinoid Hemp Oil 4200   05/17/2018

Product	SATIMED Phytocannabinoid Hemp Oil 4200
Manufacturer	SatiMed, UAB (Lithuania, European Union)
Content	Hemp Seed Oil, Full Spectrum Hemp CO2 Extract (Aerial Parts)
Use	Oral/Topical Formulations
CAS #	8016-24-8
EC #, EINECS #	289-644-3
Batch #	4
Batch Production Date	03/19/2018
Testing Sample Size	200 ml
Contacts	Email: info@satimed.eu, Tel: +370 620 33251

content → *date the test was done* *batch number* *% of cannabinoids*

General Content Values	Test Date	Test Method	Mass, %	Comment
Fats/Lipids	04/26/2018	Soxlet Method	94,15%	
Proteins (Nx6,25)	04/26/2018	Kjeldahl Method	1,25%	
Moisture	04/26/2018	SDP 5.4.4.Ch.224:2015	4,60%	

Cannabinoid Potency Values	Test Date	Test Method	Mass, %	Comment
Cannabidiol (CBD)	04/24/2018	HPLC Method	7,22%	Pass
Cannabiodiolic Acid (CBDA)	04/24/2018	HPLC Method	6,56%	Pass
Cannabigerol (CBG)	04/24/2018	HPLC Method	0,14%	
Cannabichromene (CBC)	04/24/2018	HPLC Method	0,49%	
Cannabidivarol	04/24/2018	HPLC Method	0,21%	
Cannabicitran	04/24/2018	HPLC Method	0,35%	
Cannabicyclol	04/24/2018	HPLC Method	0,07%	
Cannabinol (CBN)	04/24/2018	HPLC Method	0,01%	
Total Measured Cannabinoids	04/24/2018	HPLC Method	15,05%	Pass

total % of cannabidiol = 13.78 (round up to 14%)

14% x 30 = 4200
total cannabinoid content in 30 ML

4200 divided by 30 = 140 MG
cannabinoid content per 1 (one) ml 30 ML

there is 140 mg of CBD in each 1 ML of this product

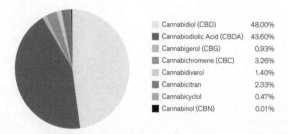

	Cannabidiol (CBD)	48.00%
	Cannabiodiolic Acid (CBDA)	43.60%
	Cannabigerol (CBG)	0.93%
	Cannabichromene (CBC)	3.26%
	Cannabidivarol	1.40%
	Cannabicitran	2.33%
	Cannabicyclol	0.47%
	Cannabinol (CBN)	0.01%

contaminants testing

 SATIMED

CERTIFICATE OF ANALYSIS

SATIMED Phytocannabinoid Hemp Oil 4200   05/17/2018

Contamination Test Results

Microbial	Date Test	Method	Mass, %	Comment
Aerobic microorganism CFU	04/27/2018	LST EN ISO 4833-1:2013	$< 1 \times 10^1$	Pass
Molds and Fungi CFU	04/27/2018	LST ISO 21527-2:2008	$< 1 \times 10^1$	Pass
Heavy Metals	**Test Date**	**Test Method**	**Mass, %**	**Comment**
Total Arsenic, mg/lg	04/27/2018	LST EN 15763:2010	nd	Pass
Total Mercury, mg/kg	04/27/2018	LST EN 15763:2010	nd	Pass
Cadmium (Cd), mg/kg	04/27/2018	LST EN 15763:2010	nd	Pass
Lead (Pb), mg/kg	04/27/2018	LST EN 15763:2010	nd	Pass
Polycyclic Aromatic Hydrocarbons by ESCH-FLD method	**Test Date**	**Test Method**	**Mass, %**	**Comment**
Sum of 4 EU PAH, μg/kg	04/27/2018	SDP 5.4.4.Ch.207:2015	nd	Pass
Benzo-a-anthracene, μg/kg	04/27/2018	SDP 5.4.4.Ch.207:2015	nd	Pass
Benzo-a-pyrene, μg/kg	04/27/2018	SDP 5.4.4.Ch.207:2015	nd	Pass
Benzo-b-fluoranthene, μg/kg	04/27/2018	SDP 5.4.4.Ch.207:2015	nd	Pass
Chrysene, μg/kg	04/27/2018	SDP 5.4.4.Ch.207:2015	nd	Pass
Pesticides	**Test Date**	**Test Method**	**Mass, %**	**Comment**
Total Pesticide Residuals by GCh-MS method, mg/kg *	04/27/2018	SDP 5.4.4.Ch.179:2014	nd	Pass
Total Pesticide Residuals by ESCh-MS/MS method, mg/kg **	04/27/2018	SDP 5.4.4.Ch.177:2013	nd	Pass

* - Total 155 Pesticides traces measured
** - Total 153 Pesticides traces measured

results = all within allowable limits

232

HEALING WITH CBD

SATIMED Phytocannabinoid Hemp Oil 4200   05/17/2018

Terpene Profile Values	Test Date	Test Method	Mass, %	Comment
β-caryophyllene	05/17/2018	GC-MS	0,746%	
tetradecanoic acid	05/17/2018	GC-MS	0,406%	
α-humulene	05/17/2018	GC-MS	0,236%	
caryophyllene oxide	05/17/2018	GC-MS	0,235%	
decanoic acid	05/17/2018	GC-MS	0,122%	
cis-β-farnesene	05/17/2018	GC-MS	0,083%	
trans-α-bergamotene	05/17/2018	GC-MS	0,080%	
β-selinene	05/17/2018	GC-MS	0,058%	
n-nonanal	05/17/2018	GC-MS	0,050%	
trans-1,3-dimethyl-cyclohexane	05/17/2018	GC-MS	0,046%	
β-pinene	05/17/2018	GC-MS	0,041%	
α-selinene	05/17/2018	GC-MS	0,037%	
ethyl-cyclohexane	05/17/2018	GC-MS	0,035%	
β-myrcene	05/17/2018	GC-MS	0,027%	
cis-1,2-dimethyl-cyclohexane	05/17/2018	GC-MS	0,024%	
octanoic acid	05/17/2018	GC-MS	0,020%	
allo-aromadendrene	05/17/2018	GC-MS	0,019%	
α-pinene	05/17/2018	GC-MS	0,019%	
nonanoic acid	05/17/2018	GC-MS	0,018%	
β-sesquiphellandrene	05/17/2018	GC-MS	0,018%	
α-zingiberene	05/17/2018	GC-MS	0,016%	
cis-caryophyllene	05/17/2018	GC-MS	0,016%	
dodecanoic acid	05/17/2018	GC-MS	0,014%	
selina-3,7(11)-diene	05/17/2018	GC-MS	0,013%	
2E-heptenal	05/17/2018	GC-MS	0,012%	
para-cymen-8-ol	05/17/2018	GC-MS	0,010%	
trans-nerolidol	05/17/2018	GC-MS	0,010%	
cis-α-bergamotene	05/17/2018	GC-MS	0,008%	
6-methyl-5-hepten-2-one	05/17/2018	GC-MS	0,004%	
terpinolene	05/17/2018	GC-MS	0,004%	

terpenes present in this batch

and their %

CONCLUSION

At the time of writing, cannabis is on the precipice of monumental and historical change. By the time you read this, it is quite possible that cannabidiol has been re-scheduled by the Drug Enforcement Agency (DEA), taking it from being heavily restricted with no recognized medicinal value to, for the first time in 80 years, being a legal compound.

While there are still many hurdles to jump, this would be HUGE news and represent progress that could not have happened without the countless patients, advocates, and educators who have worked tirelessly to move cannabis into the realm of social acceptance and availability it deserves.

And if the DEA has not rescheduled CBD, the social tides happening across the country in the form of state medical programs, adult-use legalization, and CBD-only laws mean it's only a matter of time before the federal government catches up.

It is with our sincerest hopes that you have found this book both informative and useful. Cannabis, both as a medicine and more broadly as a social movement, is a complex area, and we could have written whole books on most of the topics we've introduced here! If cannabis is important to you or a loved one, go out and learn more. We have provided resources on page 247 to help you.

And finally, we hope that cannabidiol will lead your journey to health and wellness to new heights!

Appendix

Glossary

2-AG (2-arachidonoylglycerol). An endogenous cannabinoid found in abundance in the central nervous system.

Anandamide (N-arachidonoylethanolamine or AEA). An endogenous cannabinoid named for the Sanskrit word meaning bliss (*ananda*) that works to regulate many basic bodily functions, such as appetite and sleep.

Anecdotal evidence. Evidence that comes to light through the sharing of experience between patients and their healthcare practitioners, and among themselves. While not double-blind placebo-controlled scientific research, anecdotal evidence helps inform treatment and guide research.

Antioxidant. An antioxidant is a substance, such as vitamin E, vitamin C, or beta-carotene, thought to protect body cells from the damaging effects of oxidation. The body produces its own antioxidants, and we can supplement these through diet. Cannabis is a rich source of antioxidants.

Biphasic. Literally meaning "two phases," in a medical context it means that low and high doses of the same substance can have opposite effects. Many cannabinoids have biphasic effects; for example, CBD can have alerting effects at low to moderate doses, and it can act as a sedative at high doses.

Bioaccumulation. The process by which some organisms, including cannabis and hemp, absorb and accumulate substances like pesticides and heavy metals at a faster rate than they can process and excrete them. These substances can be passed on to humans through consumption.

Bioavailability. The proportion of a drug or other substance that enters circulation when introduced into the body. Bioavailability varies depending on how the drug or substance is consumed (delivery method).

Cannabichromene (CBC). A minor cannabinoid typically found in small amounts on the cannabis plant. It is being researched for its potential to reduce pain, along with possible anti-inflammatory, antibiotic, antifungal, and anticancer effects.

Cannabidivarin (CBDV). Cannabidivarin is a non-impairing cannabinoid with a similar structure to CBD. While there is little research on CBDV, preliminary studies are showing possible antiepileptic and anti-nausea properties.

Cannabigerol (CBG). Cannabigerol is a minor cannabinoid not produced by the plant in large quantities; however, its acid form (CBGA) is the parent compound for both THCA and CBDA. CBG is a nonintoxicating cannabinoid that is useful as an antidepressant, muscle relaxant, antibiotic, antifungal agent, and blood pressure reducer.

Cannabinoid acids. As the living cannabis plant grows and develops, cannabinoids are naturally present in an acidic form. These cannabinoid acids are the molecular precursors to the more familiar cannabinoids like THC and CBD, and are converted by a process called decarboxylation. Initial research suggests that these acids, in their natural state, provide therapeutic benefits all on their own, without psychoactive effects.

HEALING with CBD

Cannabinol (CBN). Cannabinol is a by-product of the aging and oxidizing of THC. CBN is believed to have strong immunosuppressive properties, along with anti-inflammatory, antispasmodic, and antibacterial potential. At present, the relaxing and sedative properties are the main reasons consumers seek out products containing CBN.

CB1 receptor. A cannabinoid receptor found in abundance within the brain and central nervous system. The CB1 receptor is also responsible for the psychotropic effects of THC and other cannabinoids.

CB2 receptor. A cannabinoid receptor that is found in abundance within the peripheral nervous system, the immune system, and the gastrointestinal tract.

CBD-dominant/CBD-rich. In this book, we use these terms in reference to any flower or product that has higher CBD content than THC content, so anything with a CBD:THC ratio higher than 1:1.

Chemical (solvent) extraction. An extraction method by which active compounds are stripped from plant material using a solvent, often hydrocarbons (butane, propane), alcohol (ethanol), or supercritical CO_2.

Chemovar/Chemotype. In a particular species of plants, like hemp or cannabis, chemical composition varies because of different environmental growing conditions (phenotype) and/or genetics (genotype) to produce a unique chemovar or chemotype. Cannabis is often broadly divided into three large chemotype groups: Chemotype I (high THC plants), Chemotype II (balanced THC and CBD), and Chemotype III (high CBD).

Clinical Endocannabinoid Deficiency (CECD). A condition first proposed by Dr. Ethan Russo in 2004, CECD occurs when the body does not produce enough endocannabinoids or cannot regulate them properly. This can lead to illnesses that affect one or several of the bodily functions overseen by the endocannabinoid system.

Concentrates. A category of products that are characterized by a highly concentrated cannabinoid content. Historically, concentrates have been high-THC products; however, high-CBD products are being produced now as well. Concentrates are often named after their final texture: honeycomb, shatter, wax, budder, etc.

Decarboxylation. Decarboxylation is a chemical reaction that removes a carboxyl group from compounds and releases carbon dioxide. In cannabis, this process describes how the acidic forms of cannabinoids, like CBDA and THCA, are converted into CBD and THC. Decarboxylation happens when cannabis is heated, either with smoking, vaporizing, or even in the oven for use in infusions and edibles.

Delivery methods. A term used to describe the different ways in which medical cannabis can be consumed: ingestion, sublingual and mucosal, transdermal, topical, and inhalation, for example.

Dopamine. Dopamine is a neurotransmitter that helps control the brain's reward and pleasure centers. Dopamine also helps regulate movement and emotional responses—it enables us not only to see rewards, but to take action to move toward them. Dopamine deficiency results in Parkinson's disease, and people with low dopamine activity may be more prone to addiction.

HEALING with CBD

Edibles. The term used for cannabis- and hemp-based food and beverage products.

Endocannabinoids. Anandamide and 2-AG are two endogenous cannabinoids produced by the body. They act as neuromodulators to regulate various physical systems in the body.

Endocannabinoid system, or endogenous cannabinoid system (ECS). A biological system present in all mammals and many other creatures, whose purpose is to maintain balance in the body through a network of neurotransmitters, receptors, and enzymes. The endocannabinoid system helps to regulate basic bodily functions that effect how we relax, eat, sleep, forget, and protect.

Entourage effect. A theory first posited by Dr. Raphael Mechoulam in 1999 that proposes a synergistic relationship between active compounds like cannabinoids and terpenes in cannabis and hemp plants. These synergistic relationships will both change and enhance medicinal effects depending on the particular strain (or chemovar), its cannabinoid content, and its terpene profile.

Extraction method. Most cannabis- and hemp-based products are made from a concentrated extraction taken from raw plant material. Extraction can be done manually or without solvents ("solventless" extraction methods), or by using a variety of different solvents including hydrocarbons like butane or propane, alcohol like ethanol, or a pressurized form of CO_2. Each extraction method has its advantages and disadvantages for both the producer and final consumer.

First-pass metabolism. The metabolic process by which cannabinoids (or any active compounds) pass through the gastrointestinal system and are metabolized by the liver before becoming available to the body in the bloodstream. Cannabinoids that pass through the GI tract are chemically distinct and their bioavailability tends to be different from those that enter the body via other delivery methods.

Flavonoids. Flavonoids are active compounds found in cannabis and common in many plants, flowers, fruits, and vegetables. They contribute to the pigmentation, aroma, and flavor of cannabis, possibly through synergistic relationships with other active compounds like terpenes. These cannaflavins (flavonoids specific to the cannabis plant) may have medicinal properties of their own and are being studied for potential antioxidant, antifungal, and anti-inflammatory properties.

Free radicals. Unstable molecules that damage cells in the body. Too much damage can lead to oxidative stress, an imbalance that is thought to be at the root of most disease. Free radicals are produced as a by-product of normal bodily function and can also result from external sources like tobacco smoke and pesticides.

Full-spectrum. A term often used to identify products that are or were made using extracts that contain cannabinoids, terpenes, flavonoids, and other therapeutically beneficial active compounds from the cannabis plant. The active compounds in hemp and cannabis are believed to have a synergistic relationship known as "the entourage effect."

Genotype. The genetic constitution of the plant, as distinguished from the phenotype. A summary of all genetic information the plant carries and passes on to offspring.

HEALING with CBD

Glutamate. Glutamate is a neurotransmitter that is abundant in the human body, and particularly in the brain. It is an excitatory neurotransmitter that is important for neural communication, learning and memory formation.

Homeostasis. The natural state of balance in the body. Maintaining homeostasis is a dynamic process that involves all of the body's systems. The endocannabinoid system plays a vital role in achieving that balance.

Industrial hemp. Legally speaking, in the United States industrial hemp, is defined as a *Cannabis sativa* species that contains no more than 0.3% THC by dry weight. Compared to medicinal cannabis plants, industrial hemp is a far less resinous plant, but proportionally speaking, hemp contains more CBD than THC. Historically, industrial hemp has been used for its fiber and seeds.

Mechanical extraction. An extraction method by which the resin-filled trichomes on plants are physically removed, often by agitation. Kief, dry sift, and hashish are examples of products made by mechanical extraction.

Microdosing. Consuming small amounts of a medicinal compound in doses that are undetectable. In the context of cannabis- and hemp-based medicines and products, it often refers to the practice of routinely consuming small amounts of cannabinoids without experiencing impairment.

Neuroprotectants. Compounds with neuroprotective properties, like cannabinoids, reduce damage to the brain and nervous system while also encouraging the growth and development of new neurons. Neuroprotection is especially important after traumatic brain events like stroke and injury, or in the face of a neurodegenerative disease like Parkinson's or Alzheimer's.

Neurotransmitters. Chemical substances that relay messages throughout the body. Cannabinoids like THC and CBD act as neurotransmitters, as do our endogenous cannabinoids anandamide and 2-AG.

Oxidative stress. A condition that occurs when free radicals cause more damage than the body can handle. Oxidative stress is thought to be the underlying cause of many diseases.

Pharmacodynamics. The study of the biochemical and physiologic effects of drugs on the body; how a drug or active compound affects an organism.

Pharmacokinetics. The study of the bodily absorption, distribution, metabolism, and excretion of drugs and other active compounds; how an organism affects the drug or active compound.

Phenolic compounds. Phenolic compounds from medicinal herbs and dietary plants include phenolic acids, flavonoids, tannins, stilbenes, curcuminoids, coumarins, lignans, and quinones, among others. Phenolic compounds have various health benefits, including antioxidant, anticarcinogenic, antimutagenic, and anti-inflammatory effects.

Phenotype. A unique physical expression of plant genetics (genotype) as induced by its cultivation environment, which defines traits such as color, shape, smell, and resin production.

Phytocannabinoids. Cannabinoids produced by the cannabis plant, as opposed to the cannabinoids produced by the body (endocannabinoids) or synthetically.

Phytochemicals. Phytochemicals are naturally occurring chemicals produced by plants, including hemp and cannabis. Some phytochemicals (like flavonoids) give plants their pretty colors, like the blue in blueberries and the red in raspberries, and other phytochemicals (like terpenes) give plants their distinctive aromas, like basil, sage, and rosemary.

Resin. An oily substance produced by plant trichomes that contains the majority of the active compounds found in cannabis and hemp: cannabinoids, terpenoids, and flavonoids, among many others.

Self-titration. The process by which patients increase or decrease dosage themselves.

Serotonin. A neurotransmitter that impacts every part of your body, from your emotions to your motor skills. Serotonin is considered a natural mood stabilizer. It's the chemical that helps with sleeping, eating, and digesting. Too little serotonin in the brain is thought to play a role in depression.

Serotonin reuptake inhibitor. A type of drug (most often referred to as a selective serotonin reuptake inhibitor or SSRI) or compound that acts as a reuptake inhibitor of the neurotransmitter serotonin by blocking the action of the serotonin transporter. Many common prescription antidepressants work by inhibiting serotonin reuptake, and it has been shown CBD also acts to inhibit serotonin reuptake.

Spasticity. Spasticity is a condition in which certain muscles are continuously contracted. This contraction causes stiffness or tightness of the muscles and can interfere with normal movement, speech, and gait. Spasticity is usually caused by damage to the portion of the brain or spinal cord that controls voluntary movement.

Strain. Cannabis strains are either pure or hybrid varieties of the plant genus *Cannabis sativa*. Breeding has tailored the genetic makeup of plants to be high in cannabinoid content and contain specific terpenes. Strains are often named to reflect taste, color, smell, or the origin of the variety. Some varieties of *Cannabis sativa*, known as hemp, have a very low cannabinoid content and are instead grown for their fiber and seed. Hemp strains are more often referred to as "cultivars."

Sublingual delivery. Refers to the delivery method by which active compounds are absorbed by the mucosal tissue under the tongue and delivered to the bloodstream.

Terpenoids (Terpenes). Terpenes are volatile compounds found in the essential oils produced by many plants, fruits, and vegetables. Terpenes contribute to the flavor and aroma of cannabis, but also act synergistically with cannabinoids to provide a strain with its particular experiential and therapeutic profiles (see also the Entourage Effect).

Tetrahydrocannabinol (THC or delta-9-tetrahydrocannabinol). The most well-known active compound (cannabinoid) in cannabis, and often the most abundant cannabinoid in the plant. THC is responsible for many of the therapeutic effects of cannabis and produces the euphoric "high" effects cannabis is best known for.

The 2014 Farm Bill (Agricultural Act of 2014). The Agricultural Act of 2014 (aka the Farm Bill) is an omnibus legislation passed by the United States Congress and signed into law by President Obama on February 7, 2014. Under section 7606 of the Act, industrial hemp is differentiated from cannabis as long as no part of the plant (including the leaves and flowers) exceed a THC concentration of "more than 0.3 percent on a dry weight basis." Section 7606 also laid out a legal exception for growing industrial hemp in the United States under the auspices of state-approved pilot research programs.

Therapeutic window. The range of medicinal dosage that includes the minimum effective dosage up to the maximum effective dosage before side-effects become unpleasant.

Tincture. Historically, tinctures are an alcohol-based extraction, though today cannabis and hemp-based tinctures are often made from oils (hemp, MCT, avocado) that have been infused with extractions made by other methods. The traditional way of using a tincture is by sublingual absorption, though they can be added to food and drink and consumed by ingestion as well.

Topicals. The term used for cannabis and hemp-based creams, salves, balms, and any product that you apply locally to the skin.

Transdermal delivery. Refers to the delivery method by which active compounds are absorbed by all layers of the skin (derma) and enter the bloodstream.

Trichomes. Trichomes are tiny glandular hairs that develop on the surface of cannabis and hemp plants, particularly on the upper leaves and flowers. It is within these trichomes that the oily mixture (resin) containing active compounds like cannabinoids, terpenoids (terpenes), flavonoids, and other phytochemicals is produced and stored.

Whole-plant. A term often used to identify products that are or were made using extracts that contain cannabinoids, terpenes, flavonoids, and other therapeutically beneficial active compounds from the cannabis plant. The active compounds in hemp and cannabis are believed to have a synergistic relationship known as "the entourage effect."

Medical Cannabis Log

Date:_____

Symptoms/Needs: _____

_____

_____

_____

_____

Pre-treatment pain level (indicate on a 1-10 scale): _____

Method of delivery: _____

Product Details:_____

Dosage: _____

Terpenes/Cannabinoids: _____

Effects: _____

Post-treatment pain level (indicate on a 1-10 scale): _____

Would you use this product again? Explain:_____

_____

_____

Additional Notes: _____

_____

_____

_____

Resources

Books

CBD: A Patient's Guide to Medical Cannabis—Healing Without the High by Leonard Leinow and Juliana Birnbaum

Cannabis for Chronic Pain: A Proven Prescription for Using Marijuana to Relieve Your Pain and Heal Your Life by Dr. Rav Ivker

The Cannabis Health Index: Combining the Science of Medical Marijuana with Mindfulness Techniques To Heal 100 Chronic Symptoms and Diseases by Uwe Blesching

Cannabis Pharmacy: The Practical Guide to Medical Marijuana by Michael Backes

Cannabis Revealed: How the World's Most Misunderstood Plant is Healing Everything from Chronic Pain to Epilepsy by Dr. Bonni Goldstein

The Leafly Guide to Cannabis: A Handbook for the Modern Consumer by The Leafly Team

The Pot Book: A Complete Guide to Cannabis edited by Dr. Julie Holland

Smoke Signals: A Social History of Marijuana—Medical, Recreational and Scientific by Martin A. Lee

Stoned: A Doctor's Case for Medical Marijuana by David Casarett, MD

General Online Resources

Project CBD, https://www.projectcbd.org

CBD School, https://cbdschool.com

Olive's Branch, http://www.olives-branch.com

Green Flower, https://www.green-flower.com

Prof of Pot, http://profofpot.com

Medical Jane, https://www.medicaljane.com

Ministry of Hemp, https://ministryofhemp.com

Leaf Science, https://www.leafscience.com

O'Shaughnessy's, http://www.beyondthc.com

Americans for Safe Access, https://www.safeaccessnow.org/resources_for_patients

United Patients Group, https://unitedpatientsgroup.com

Leafly, https://www.leafly.com

Scientific Research

Pub Med, https://www.ncbi.nlm.nih.gov/pubmed

ClinicalTrials.gov, https://www.clinicaltrials.gov

The International Cannabinoid Research Society, http://icrs.co

Finding a Doctor or Healthcare Practitioner

Association of Cannabis Specialists, https://www.cannabis-specialists.org/directory-of-specialists

Society of Cannabis Clinicians, http://cannabisclinicians.org/referrals

American Cannabis Nurses Association, https://cannabisnurses.org

Notes

1   Vincenzo Di Marzo and Fabiana Piscitelli, "The Endocannabinoid System and Its Modulation by Phytocannabinoids," *Neurotherapeutics* 12, no. 4 (2015): 692–98, doi:10.1007/s13311-015-0374-6.

2   Daniel R. McDougle et al., "Anti-Inflammatory ω-3 Endocannabinoid Epoxides," *Proceedings of the National Academy of Sciences* 114, no. 30 (2017), doi:10.1073/pnas.1610325114.

3   John M. McPartland et al., "Care and Feeding of the Endocannabinoid System: A Systematic Review of Potential Clinical Interventions That Upregulate the Endocannabinoid System," *PLoS One* 9, no. 3 (2014), doi:10.1371/journal.pone.0089566.

4   McPartland et al., "Care and Feeding."

5   Maria Morena et al., "Neurobiological Interactions between Stress and the Endocannabinoid System," *Neuropsychopharmacology* 41, no. 1 (2016): 80–102, doi:10.1038/npp.2015.166.

6   Elsa Heyman et al., "Intense Exercise Increases Circulating Endocannabinoid and BDNF Levels in Humans—Possible Implications for Reward and Depression," *Psychoneuroendocrinology* 37, no. 6 (2012): 844–51, doi:10.1016/j.psyneuen.2011.09.017.

7   Raymond Niesink et al., "Does Cannabidiol Protect Against Adverse Psychological Effects of THC?", *Frontiers in Psychiatry* 4, no. 4 (2013): 130, doi:10.3389/fpsyt.2013.00130.

8   J. D. Wilkinson et al., "Medicinal Cannabis: Is Δ9-Tetrahydrocannabinol Necessary for All Its Effects?" *Journal of Pharmacy and Pharmacology* 55, no. 12 (2004): 1687–94, doi:10.1211/0022357022304.

9   Angélica Maria Sabogal-Guáqueta, Edison Osorio, and Gloria Patricia Cardona-Gómez, "Linalool Reverses Neuropathological and Behavioral Impairments in Old Triple Transgenic Alzheimers Mice," *Neuropharmacology* 102, (2016): 111–20, doi:10.1016/j.neuropharm.2015.11.002.

10   A. L. Klauke et al., "The Cannabinoid CB2 Receptor-Selective Phytocannabinoid Beta-Caryophyllene Exerts Analgesic Effects in Mouse Models of Inflammatory and Neuropathic Pain," *European Neuropsychopharmacology* 24, no. 4 (2014): 608–20, doi:10.1016/j.euroneuro.2013.10.008.

11   Amine Bahi et al., "β-Caryophyllene, a CB2 Receptor Agonist Produces Multiple Behavioral Changes Relevant to Anxiety and Depression in Mice," *Physiology & Behavior* 135, (2014): 119–24, doi:10.1016/j.physbeh.2014.06.003.

12   T. G. do Vale et al., "Central Effects of Citral, Myrcene and Limonene, Constituents of Essential Oil Chemotypes from Lippia Alba (Mill.) N.E. Brown," *Phytomedicine* 9, no. 8 (2002): 709–14.

13   V. S. Rao, A. M. Menezes, and G. S. Viana, "Effect of Myrcene on Nociception in Mice," *Journal of Pharmacy and Pharmacology* 42, no. 12 (1990): 877–78, doi:10.1111/j.2042-7158.1990.tb07046.x.; L. I. Paula-Freire et al., "Evaluation of the Antinociceptive Activity Of Ocimum GratissimumL. (Lamiaceae) Essential Oil and Its Isolated Active Principles in Mice," *Phytotherapy Research* 27, no. 8 (2013): 1220–24, doi:10.1002/ptr.4845.

14   Aline De Moraes Pultrini, Luciane Almeida Galindo, and Mirtes Costa, "Effects of the Essential Oil from Citrus Aurantium L. in Experimental Anxiety Models in Mice," *Life Sciences* 78, no. 15 (2006): 1720–25, doi:10.1016/j.lfs.2005.08.004.

15   C. F. Zhang, Z. L. Yang, and J. B. Luo, "Effects of D-Limonene and L-Limonene on Transdermal Absorption of Ligustrazine Hydrochloride," *Yao Xue Xue Bao* 41, no. 8 (2006): 772–77.

16   J. Sun, "D-Limonene: Safety and Clinical Applications," *Alternative Medicine Review* 12, no. 3 (2007): 259–64.

17   R. L. Jirtle et al., "Increased Mannose 6-Phosphate/Insulin-like Growth Factor II Receptor and Transforming Growth Factor Beta 1 Levels during Monoterpene-Induced Regression of Mammary Tumors," *Cancer Research* 53, no. 17 (1993): 3849–52.

18 M. G. de Oliveira et al., "α-Terpineol Reduces Mechanical Hypernociception and Inflammatory Response," *Basic & Clinical Pharmacology & Toxicology* 111, no. 2 (2012): 120–25, doi:10.1111/j.1742-7843.2012.00875.x.

19 R. H. L. Souza et al., "Gastroprotective Activity of α-Terpineol in Two Experimental Models of Gastric Ulcer in Rats," *DARU Journal of Pharmaceutical Sciences* 19, no. 4 (2011): 277–81.

20 Li Li et al., "Antibacterial Activity of a-Terpineol May Induce Morphostructural Alterations in Escherichia Coli," *Brazilian Journal of Microbiology* 45, no. 4 (2015): 1409–13, doi:10.1590/s1517-83822014000400035.

21 J. L. Bicas et al., "Evaluation of the Antioxidant and Antiproliferative Potential of Bioflavors," *Food and Chemical Toxicology* 49, no. 7 (2011): 1610–15, doi:10.1016/j.fct.2011.04.012.

22 A. J. Hampson et al., "Cannabidiol and (−)Δ⁹-Tetrahydro-cannabinol Are Neuroprotective Antioxidants," *Proceedings of the National Academy of Sciences* 95, no. 14 (1998): 8268–73, doi:10.1073/pnas.95.14.8268.

23 Kerstin Iffland and Franjo Grotenhermen, "An Update on Safety and Side Effects of Cannabidiol: A Review of Clinical Data and Relevant Animal Studies," *Cannabis and Cannabinoid Research* 2, no. 1 (2017): 139–54, doi:10.1089/can.2016.0034.

24 M. M. Bergamaschi et al., "Safety and Side Effects of Cannabidiol, a Cannabis Sativa Constituent," *Current Drug Safety* 6, no. 4 (2011): 237–49, doi:10.2174/157488611798280924.

25 Amanda Reiman, Mark Welty, and Perry Solomon, "Cannabis as a Substitute for Opioid-Based Pain Medication: Patient Self-Report," *Cannabis and Cannabinoid Research* 2, no. 1 (2017): 160–66, doi:10.1089/can.2017.0012.

26 Kevin F. Boehnke, Evangelos Litinas, and Daniel J. Clauw, "Medical Cannabis Use Is Associated with Decreased Opiate Medication Use in a Retrospective Cross-Sectional Survey of Patients

with Chronic Pain," *The Journal of Pain* 17, no. 6 (2016): 739–44, doi:10.1016/j.jpain.2016.03.002.

27   Gustavo Gonzalez-Cuevas et al., "Unique Treatment Potential of Cannabidiol for the Prevention of Relapse to Drug Use: Preclinical Proof of Principle," *Neuropsychopharmacology* (2018), doi:10.1038/s41386-018-0050-8.

28   Kerstin Iffland and Franjo Grotenhermen, "An Update on Safety and Side Effects of Cannabidiol: A Review of Clinical Data and Relevant Animal Studies," *Cannabis and Cannabinoid Research* 2, no. 1 (2017): 139–54, doi:10.1089/can.2016.0034.

29   E. L. Gardner, "Endocannabinoid Signaling System and Brain Reward: Emphasis on Dopamine," *Pharmacology Biochemistry and Behavior* 81, no. 2 (2005): 263–84, doi:10.1016/j.pbb.2005.01.032.

30   Daniel Liput et al., "Transdermal Delivery of Cannabidiol Attenuates Binge Alcohol-Induced Neurodegeneration in a Rodent Model of an Alcohol Use Disorder," *Pharmacology Biochemistry and Behavior* 111 (2013): 120-127, doi:/10.1016/j.pbb.2013.08.013.

31   Yuping Wang et al., "Cannabidiol Attenuates Alcohol-Induced Liver Steatosis, Metabolic Dysregulation, Inflammation and Neutrophil-Mediated Injury," *Scientific Reports* 7, no. 1 (2017), doi:10.1038/s41598-017-10924-8.

32   Gustavo Gonzalez-Cuevas et al., "Unique Treatment Potential of Cannabidiol for the Prevention of Relapse to Drug Use: Preclinical Proof of Principle," *Neuropsychopharmacology* (2018), doi:10.1038/s41386-018-0050-8.

33   Chandni Hindocha et al., "Cannabidiol Reverses Attentional Bias to Cigarette Cues in a Human Experimental Model of Tobacco Withdrawal," *Addiction*, May (2018), doi:10.1111/add.14243.

34   Yasmin L. Hurd et al., "Early Phase in the Development of Cannabidiol as a Treatment for Addiction: Opioid Relapse Takes Initial Center Stage," *Neurotherapeutics* 12, no. 4 (2015): 807–15, doi:10.1007/s13311-015-0373-7.

35   Yanhua Ren et al., "Cannabidiol, a Nonpsychotropic Component of Cannabis, Inhibits Cue-Induced Heroin Seeking and Normalizes Discrete Mesolimbic Neuronal Disturbances," *Journal of Neuroscience* 29, no. 47 (2010): 14764–69, doi:10.1523/jneurosci.4291-09.2009.

36   Thangavelu Soundara Rajan et al., "Gingival Stromal Cells as an In Vitro Model: Cannabidiol Modulates Genes Linked with Amyotrophic Lateral Sclerosis," *Journal of Cellular Biochemistry* 118, no. 4 (2016): 819–28, doi:10.1002/jcb.25757.

37   Gregory T. Carter et al., "Cannabis and Amyotrophic Lateral Sclerosis: Hypothetical and Practical Applications, and a Call for Clinical Trials," *American Journal of Hospice and Palliative Medicine* 27, no. 5 (2010): 347–56, doi:10.1177/1049909110369531.

38   Emanuela Mazzon and Sabrina Giacoppo, "Can Cannabinoids Be a Potential Therapeutic Tool in Amyotrophic Lateral Sclerosis?" *Neural Regeneration Research* 11, no. 12 (2016): 1896–99, doi:10.4103/1673-5374.197125.

39   Rajan et al., "Gingival Stromal Cells as an In Vitro Model," 819–28.

40   A. Calignano et al., "Bidirectional Control of Airway Responsiveness by Endogenous Cannabinoids," *Nature* 408, no. 6808 (2000): 96–101.

41   Sumner Burstein, "Cannabidiol (CBD) and Its Analogs: a Review of Their Effects on Inflammation," *Bioorganic & Medicinal Chemistry* 23, no. 7 (2015): 1377–85, doi:10.1016/j.bmc.2015.01.059.

42   Francieli Vuolo et al., "Evaluation of Serum Cytokines Levels and the Role of Cannabidiol Treatment in Animal Model of Asthma," *Mediators of Inflammation* 2015, (May 2015). doi:10.1155/2015/538670.

43   C. Földy, R. C. Malenka, and T. C. Südhof, "Autism-Associated Neuroligin-3 Mutations Commonly Disrupt Tonic Endocannabinoid Signaling," *Neuron* 78, no. 3 (2013): 498–509, doi:10.1016/j.neuron.2013.02.036.

44   Dario Siniscalco et al., "Cannabinoid Receptor Type 2, but Not Type 1, Is Up-Regulated in Peripheral Blood Mononuclear Cells of

Children Affected by Autistic Disorders," *Journal of Autism and Developmental Disorders* 43, no. 11 (2013): 2686–95, doi:10.1007/s10803-013-1824-9.

45   V. M. Doenni et al., "Deficient Adolescent Social Behavior Following Early-Life Inflammation Is Ameliorated by Augmentation of Anandamide Signaling," *Brain, Behavior, and Immunity* 58 (July 2016): 237–47, doi:10.1016/j.bbi.2016.07.152.

46   Georgia Watt and Tim Karl, "*In vivo* Evidence for Therapeutic Properties of Cannabidiol (CBD) for Alzheimers Disease," *Frontiers in Pharmacology* 8 (February 2017): 20, doi:10.3389/fphar.2017.00020.

47   A. M. Martín-Moreno et al., "Cannabidiol and Other Cannabinoids Reduce Microglial Activation In Vitro and In Vivo: Relevance to Alzheimers Disease," *Molecular Pharmacology* 79, no. 6 (2011): 964–73, doi:10.1124/mol.111.071290.

48   David Cheng et al., "Long-Term Cannabidiol Treatment Prevents the Development of Social Recognition Memory Deficits in Alzheimers Disease Transgenic Mice," *Journal of Alzheimers Disease* 42, no. 4 (2014): 1383–96, doi:10.3233/jad-140921.

49   Melanie-Jayne R. Howes and Elaine Perry, "The Role of Phytochemicals in the Treatment and Prevention of Dementia," *Drugs & Aging* 28, no. 6 (2011): 439–68, doi:10.2165/11591310-000000000-00000.

50   Peter Strohbeck-Huehner, Gisela Skopp, and Tainer Mattern, "Cannabis Improves Symptoms of ADHD," *Cannabinoids* 3, no. 1 (2008): 1–3.

51   Maura Castelli et al., "Loss of Striatal Cannabinoid CB1 Receptor Function in Attention-Deficit/Hyperactivity Disorder Mice with Point-Mutation of the Dopamine Transporter," *European Journal of Neuroscience* 43, no. 9 (2011): 1369-1377, doi:10.1111/j.1460-9568.2011.07876.x.

52   Esther M. Blessing et al., "Cannabidiol as a Potential Treatment for Anxiety Disorders," *Neurotherapeutics* 12, no. 4 (2015): 825–36, doi:10.1007/s13311-015-0387-1.

53   Raquel Linge et al., "Cannabidiol Induces Rapid-Acting Antidepressant-like Effects and Enhances Cortical 5-HT/Glutamate Neurotransmission: Role of 5-HT1A Receptors," *Neuropharmacology* 103, (December 2015): 16–26, doi:10.1016/j.neuropharm.2015.12.017.

54   Alline C. Campos et al., "The Anxiolytic Effect of Cannabidiol on Chronically Stressed Mice Depends on Hippocampal Neurogenesis: Involvement of the Endocannabinoid System," *The International Journal of Neuropsychopharmacology* 16, no. 6 (2013): 1407–19, doi:10.1017/s1461145712001502.

55   José Alexandre S. Crippa et al., "Neural Basis of Anxiolytic Effects of Cannabidiol (CBD) in Generalized Social Anxiety Disorder: a Preliminary Report," *Journal of Psychopharmacology* 25, no. 1 (2010): 121–30, doi:10.1177/0269881110379283.

56   Mateus M. Bergamaschi et al., "Cannabidiol Reduces the Anxiety Induced by Simulated Public Speaking in Treatment-Naïve Social Phobia Patients," *Neuropsychopharmacology* 36, no. 6 (2011): 1219–26.

57   Leonardo B. M. Resstel et al., "5-HT1A Receptors Are Involved in the Cannabidiol-Induced Attenuation of Behavioural and Cardiovascular Responses to Acute Restraint Stress in Rats," *British Journal of Pharmacology* 156, no. 1 (2009): 181–88, doi:10.1111/j.1476-5381.2008.00046.x.

58   Mark A. Lewis, Ethan B. Russo, and Kevin M. Smith, "Pharmacological Foundations of Cannabis Chemovars," *Planta Medica* 84, no. 4 (2017): 225–33, doi:10.1055/s-0043-122240.

59   Ethan B. Russo, "Taming THC: Potential Cannabis Synergy and Phytocannabinoid-Terpenoid Entourage Effects," *British Journal of Pharmacology* 163, no. 7 (2011): 1344–64, doi:10.1111/j.1476-5381.2011.01238.x.

60   Sumner Burstein, "Cannabidiol (CBD) and Its Analogs: a Review of Their Effects on Inflammation," *Bioorganic & Medicinal Chemistry* 23, no. 7 (2015): 1377–85, doi:10.1016/j.bmc.2015.01.059.

61   Carmen La Porta et al., "Involvement of the Endocannabinoid System in Osteoarthritis Pain," *European Journal of Neuroscience* 39, no. 3 (2014): 485–500, doi:10.1111/ejn.12468.

62   D. C. Hammell et al., "Transdermal Cannabidiol Reduces Inflammation and Pain-Related Behaviours in a Rat Model of Arthritis," *European Journal of Pain* 20, no. 6 (2015): 936–48, doi:10.1002/ejp.818.

63   A. M. Malfait et al., "The Nonpsychoactive Cannabis Constituent Cannabidiol Is an Oral Anti-Arthritic Therapeutic in Murine Collagen-Induced Arthritis," *Proceedings of the National Academy of Sciences* 97, no. 17 (2000): 9561–66, doi:10.1073/pnas.160105897.

64   D. R. Blake et al., "Preliminary Assessment of the Efficacy, Tolerability and Safety of a Cannabis-Based Medicine (Sativex) in the Treatment of Pain Caused by Rheumatoid Arthritis," *Rheumatology* 45, no. 1 (2005): 50–52, doi:10.1093/rheumatology/kei183.

65   George W. Booz, "Cannabidiol as an Emergent Therapeutic Strategy for Lessening the Impact of Inflammation on Oxidative Stress," *Free Radical Biology and Medicine* 51, no. 5 (2011): 1054–61, doi:10.1016/j.freeradbiomed.2011.01.007.

66   P. Pacher, S. Bátkai, and G. Kunos, "The Endocannabinoid System as an Emerging Target of Pharmacotherapy," *Pharmacological Reviews* 58, no. 3 (2008): 389–462, doi:10.1124/pr.58.3.2.

67   G. A. Cabral and A. Staab, "Effects on the Immune System," *Handbook of Experimental Pharmacology Cannabinoids*, no. 168 (2005): 385–423, doi:10.1007/3-540-26573-2_13.

68   Prakash Nagarkatti et al., "Cannabinoids as Novel Anti-Inflammatory Drugs," *Future Medicinal Chemistry* 1, no. 7 (2009): 1333–49, doi:10.4155/fmc.09.93.

69   Lola Weiss et al., "Cannabidiol Arrests Onset of Autoimmune Diabetes in NOD Mice," *Neuropharmacology* 54, no. 1 (2009): 244–49, doi:10.1016/j.neuropharm.2007.06.029.

70   Paola Massi et al., "Cannabidiol as Potential Anticancer Drug," *British Journal of Clinical Pharmacology* 75 no. 2 (2013): 303–12, doi:10.1111/j.1365-2125.2012.04298.x.

71   Massi, "Cannabidiol as Potential Anticancer Drug," 303–12.

72   M. Solinas et al., "Cannabidiol Inhibits Angiogenesis by Multiple Mechanisms," *British Journal of Pharmacology* 167, no. 6 (2012): 1218–31, doi:10.1111/j.1476-5381.2012.02050.x.

73   A.I. Fraguas-Sanchez, A. Fernandez-Carballido, and A.I. Torres-Suarez, "Phyto-, endo-, and synthetic cannabinoids: promising chemotherapeutic agents in the treatment of breast and prostate carcinomas," Expert Opinion on *Investigational Drugs* 25, no. 11 (2016): 1311-1323, doi:10.1080/13543784.2016.1236913.

74   Sean D. McAllister, Liliana Soroceanu, and Pierre-Yves Desprez, "The Antitumor Activity of Plant-Derived Non-Psychoactive Cannabinoids," *Journal of Neuroimmune Pharmacology* 10, no. 2 (2015): 255–67, doi:10.1007/s11481-015-9608-y.

75   Katherine Ann Scott et al., "Enhancing the Activity of Cannabidiol and Other Cannabinoids *In Vitro* Through Modifications to Drug Combinations and Treatment Schedules," *Anticancer Research* 33, no. 10 (2013): 4373–80.

76   Dereck T. Wade et al., "A Preliminary Controlled Study to Determine Whether Whole-Plant Cannabis Extracts Can Improve Intractable Neurogenic Symptoms," *Clinical Rehabilitation* 17, no. 1 (2003): 21–29, doi:10.1191/0269215503cr581oa.

77   Marcelo Kwiatkoski, Francisco Silveira Guimarães, and Elaine Del-Bel, "Cannabidiol-Treated Rats Exhibited Higher Motor Score After Cryogenic Spinal Cord Injury," *Neurotoxicity Research* 21, no. 3 (2011): 271–80, doi:10.1007/s12640-011-9273-8.

78   David Fernández-López et al., "Cannabinoids: Well-Suited Candidates for the Treatment of Perinatal Brain Injury," *Brain Sciences* 3, no. 3 (2013): 1043–59, doi:10.3390/brainsci3031043.

79   Matthew N. Hill et al., "Regional Alterations in the Endocannabinoid System in an Animal Model of Depression:

Effects of Concurrent Antidepressant Treatment," *Journal of Neurochemistry* 106, no. 6 (2008): 2322–36, doi:10.1111/j.1471-4159.2008.05567.x.

80   Raquel Linge et al., "Cannabidiol Induces Rapid-Acting Antidepressant-like Effects and Enhances Cortical 5-HT/Glutamate Neurotransmission: Role of 5-HT1A Receptors," *Neuropharmacology* 103, (December 2015): 16–26, doi:10.1016/j.neuropharm.2015.12.017.

81   Béla Horváth et al., "The Endocannabinoid System and Plant-Derived Cannabinoids in Diabetes and Diabetic Complications," *The American Journal of Pathology* 180, no. 2 (2012): 432–42, doi:10.1016/j.ajpath.2011.11.003.

82   Khalid A. Jadoon et al., "Efficacy and Safety of Cannabidiol and Tetrahydrocannabivarin on Glycemic and Lipid Parameters in Patients With Type 2 Diabetes: A Randomized, Double-Blind, Placebo-Controlled, Parallel Group Pilot Study," *Diabetes Care* 39, no. 10 (2016): 1777–86, doi:10.2337/dc16-0650.

83   Mohanraj Rajesh et al., "Cannabidiol Attenuates High Glucose-Induced Endothelial Cell Inflammatory Response and Barrier Disruption," *American Journal of Physiology-Heart and Circulatory Physiology* 293, no. 1 (2007): H610–H619, doi:10.1152/ajpheart.00236.2007.

84   Lola Weiss et al., "Cannabidiol Arrests Onset of Autoimmune Diabetes in NOD Mice," *Neuropharmacology* 54, no. 1 (2009): 244–49, doi:10.1016/j.neuropharm.2007.06.029.

85   L. Weiss et al., "Cannabidiol Arrests," 2006.

86   Azza B. El-Remessy et al., "Neuroprotective and Blood-Retinal Barrier-Preserving Effects of Cannabidiol in Experimental Diabetes," *The American Journal of Pathology* 168, no. 1 (2006): 235–44, doi:10.2353/ajpath.2006.050500.

87   Brian Walitt et al., "Cannabinoids for Fibromyalgia," *Cochrane Database of Systematic Reviews* 7, (July 2016), doi:10.1002/14651858.cd011694.pub2.

88   George Habib and Suheil Artul, "Medical Cannabis for the Treatment of Fibromyalgia," *JCR: Journal of Clinical Rheumatology* 24, no. 5 (2018): 255–58, doi:10.1097/rhu.0000000000000702.

89   Angelo A. Izzo and Keith B. Sharkey, "Cannabinoids and the Gut: New Developments and Emerging Concepts," *Pharmacology & Therapeutics* 126, no. 1 (2010): 21–38, doi:10.1016/j.pharmthera.2009.12.005.

90   Haidar Shamran et al., "Fatty Acid Amide Hydrolase (FAAH) Blockade Ameliorates Experimental Colitis by Altering MicroRNA Expression and Suppressing Inflammation," *Brain, Behavior, and Immunity* 59 (June 2016): 10–20, doi:10.1016/j.bbi.2016.06.008.

91   R. Capasso et al., "Cannabidiol, Extracted From *Cannabis sativa*, Selectively Inhibits Inflammatory Hypermotility in Mice," *British Journal of Pharmacology* 154, no. 5 (2008): 1001–8, doi:10.1038/bjp.2008.177.

92   Giuseppe Esposito et al., "Cannabidiol in Inflammatory Bowel Diseases: A Brief Overview," *Phytotherapy Research* 27, no. 5 (2012): 633–36, doi:10.1002/ptr.4781.

93   J. M. Jamontt et al., "The Effects of Δ9-Tetrahydrocannabinol and Cannabidiol Alone and in Combination on Damage, Inflammation Andin Vitromotility Disturbances in Rat Colitis," *British Journal of Pharmacology* 160, no. 3 (2010): 712–23, doi:10.1111/j.1476-5381.2010.00791.x.

94   Daniele De Filippis et al., "Cannabidiol Reduces Intestinal Inflammation through the Control of Neuroimmune Axis," *PLoS ONE* 6, no. 12 (2011), doi:10.1371/journal.pone.0028159.

95   Ethan B. Russo, "Clinical Endocannabinoid Deficiency (CECD): Can This Concept Explain Therapeutic Benefits of Cannabis in Migraine, Fibromyalgia, Irritable Bowel Syndrome and Other Treatment-Resistant Conditions?" *Neuro Endocrinology Letters* 29, no. 2 (2008): 192–200.

96   Russo, "Clinical Endocannabinoid Deficiency," 192–200.

97   Ethan B. Russo, "Cannabinoids in the Management of Difficult to Treat Pain," *Therapeutics and Clinical Risk Management* 4, no. 1 (2008): 245–59, doi:10.2147/tcrm.s1928.

98   Rosaria Greco et al., "Activation of CB2 Receptors as a Potential Therapeutic Target for Migraine: Evaluation in an Animal Model," *The Journal of Headache and Pain* 15, no. 1 (2014): 14, doi:10.1186/1129-2377-15-14.

99   "Cannabinoids Suitable for Migraine Prevention," *EAN*, EAN, European Academy of Neurology, (2017) https://www.ean.org/amsterdam2017/fileadmin/user_upload/E-EAN_2017_-_Cannabinoids_in_migraine_-_FINAL.pdf.

100   David Baker et al., "The Biology That Underpins the Therapeutic Potential of Cannabis-Based Medicines for the Control of Spasticity in Multiple Sclerosis," *Multiple Sclerosis and Related Disorders* 1, no. 2 (2012): 64–75, doi:10.1016/j.msard.2011.11.001.

101   S. Giacoppo et al., "Purified Cannabidiol, the Main Non-Psychotropic Component of Cannabis Sativa, Alone, Counteracts Neuronal Apoptosis in Experimental Multiple Sclerosis," *European Review for Medical and Pharmacological Sciences* 19, no. 24 (2015): 4906–19.

102   Varda Mei-Tal, Sanford Meyerowitz, and George L. Engel, "The Role of Psychological Process in a Somatic Disorder: Multiple Sclerosis," *Psychosomatic Medicine* 32, no. 1 (1970): 67–86, doi:10.1097/00006842-197001000-00006.

103   K. D. Ackerman et al., "Stressful Life Events Precede Exacerbations of Multiple Sclerosis," *Psychosomatic Medicine* 64, no. 6 (2002): 916–20, doi:10.1097/01.psy.0000038941.33335.40.

104   E. M. Rock et al., "Cannabidiol, a Non-Psychotropic Component of Cannabis, Attenuates Vomiting and Nausea-like Behaviour via Indirect Agonism of 5-HT1A Somatodendritic Autoreceptors in the Dorsal Raphe Nucleus," *British Journal of Pharmacology* 165, no. 8 (2012): 2620–34, doi:10.1111/j.1476-5381.2011.01621.x.

105 E. M. Rock et al., "Cannabinoid Regulation of Acute and Anticipatory Nausea," *Cannabis and Cannabinoid Research* 1, no. 1 (2016): 113–21, doi:10.1089/can.2016.0006.

106 D. Bolognini et al., "Cannabidiolic Acid Prevents Vomiting InSuncus Murinusand Nausea-Induced Behaviour in Rats by Enhancing 5-HT1A receptor Activation," *British Journal of Pharmacology* 168, no. 6 (2013): 1456–70, doi:10.1111/bph.12043.

107 L. D. O'Brien et al., "Anandamide Transport Inhibition by ARN272 Attenuates Nausea-Induced Behaviour in Rats, and Vomiting in Shrews (Suncus Murinus)," *British Journal of Pharmacology* 170, no. 5 (2013): 1130–36, doi:10.1111/bph.12360.

108 Hilal Ahmad Parray and Jong Won Yun, "Cannabidiol Promotes Browning in 3T3-L1 Adipocytes," *Molecular and Cellular Biochemistry* 416, no. 1–2 (2016): 131–39, doi:10.1007/s11010-016-2702-5.

109 Itay Lotan et al., "Cannabis (Medical Marijuana) Treatment for Motor and Non–Motor Symptoms of Parkinson Disease," *Clinical Neuropharmacology* 37, no. 2 (2014): 41–44, doi:10.1097/wnf.0000000000000016.

110 Sandeep Vasant More and Dong-Kug Choi, "Promising Cannabinoid-Based Therapies for Parkinson's Disease: Motor Symptoms to Neuroprotection," *Molecular Neurodegeneration* 10, (April 2015): 17, doi:10.1186/s13024-015-0012-0.

111 Sandeep Vasant More and Dong-Kug Choi, "Emerging Preclinical Pharmacological Targets for Parkinson's Disease," *Oncotarget* 7, no. 20 (2016): 29835–63, doi:10.18632/oncotarget.8104.

112 Marcos Hortes N. Chagas et al., "Effects of Cannabidiol in the Treatment of Patients with Parkinson's Disease: An Exploratory Double-Blind Trial," *Journal of Psychopharmacology* 28, no. 11 (2014): 1088–98, doi:10.1177/0269881114550355.

113 Teresa Iuvone et al, "Cannabidiol: A Promising Drug for Neurodegenerative Disorders?" *CNS Neuroscience & Therapeutics* 15, no. 1 (2009): 65-75, doi: 10.1111/j.1755-5949.2008.00065.x.

114   Rosaria Greco et al., "The Endocannabinoid System and Migraine," *Experimental Neurology* 224, no. 1 (2010): 85–91, doi:10.1016/j.expneurol.2010.03.029.

115   Ethan B. Russo, "Cannabinoids in the Management of Difficult to Treat Pain," *Therapeutics and Clinical Risk Management* 4, no. 1 (2008): 245–59, doi:10.2147/tcrm.s1928.

116   Kevin F. Boehnke, Evangelos Litinas, and Daniel J. Clauw, "Medical Cannabis Use Is Associated with Decreased Opiate Medication Use in a Retrospective Cross-Sectional Survey of Patients with Chronic Pain," *The Journal of Pain* 17, no. 6 (2016): 739–44, doi:10.1016/j.jpain.2016.03.002.

117   Ethan B. Russo and Andrea G Hohmann, "Role of Cannabinoids in Pain Management," Essay, In *Treatment of Chronic Pain by Medical Approaches*, (2013): 181–97. New York, NY: Springer.

118   Jeremy R. Johnson et al., "Multicenter, Double-Blind, Randomized, Placebo-Controlled, Parallel-Group Study of the Efficacy, Safety, and Tolerability of THC:CBD Extract and THC Extract in Patients with Intractable Cancer-Related Pain," *Journal of Pain and Symptom Management* 39, no. 2 (2009): 167–79, doi:10.1016/j.jpainsymman.2009.06.008.

119   D. I. Abrams and M. Guzman, "Cannabis in Cancer Care," *Clinical Pharmacology and Therapeutics* 97, no. 6 (2015): 575–86, doi:0.1002/cpt.108.

120   Jonathan L. C. Lee et al., "Cannabidiol Regulation of Emotion and Emotional Memory Processing: Relevance for Treating Anxiety-Related and Substance Abuse Disorders," *British Journal of Pharmacology* 174, no. 19 (2017): 3242–56, doi:10.1111/bph.13724.

121   Chenchen Song, et al., "Bidirectional Effects of Cannabidiol on Contextual Fear Memory Extinction," *Frontiers in Pharmacology* 16, no. 7 (2016), doi:10.3389/fphar.2016.00493.

122   Matthew N. Hill et al., "Reductions in Circulating Endo-cannabinoid Levels in Individuals with Post-Traumatic Stress Disorder Following Exposure to the World Trade Center Attacks,"

Psychoneuroendocrinology 38, no. 12 (2013): 2952–61, doi:10.1016/j.psyneuen.2013.08.004.

123 Tabitha A. Iseger and Matthijs G. Bossong, "A Systematic Review of the Antipsychotic Properties of Cannabidiol in Humans," *Schizophrenia Research* 162, no. 1–3 (2015): 153–61, doi:10.1016/j.schres.2015.01.033.

124 A.W. Zuardi et al., "Cannabidiol, a Cannabis Sativa Constituent, as an Antipsychotic Drug," *Brazilian Journal of Medical and Biological Research* 39, no. 4 (2006): 421–29, doi:10.1590/s0100-879x2006000400001.

125 Ethan B. Russo, "Clinical Endocannabinoid Deficiency (CECD): Can This Concept Explain Therapeutic Benefits of Cannabis in Migraine, Fibromyalgia, Irritable Bowel Syndrome and Other Treatment-Resistant Conditions?" *Neuro Endocrinology Letters* 25, no. 1–2 (2004): 31–39.

126 Chung Mo Koo and Hoon-Chul Kang, "Could Cannabidiol Be a Treatment Option for Intractable Childhood and Adolescent Epilepsy?" *Journal of Epilepsy Research* 7, no. 1 (2017): 16–20, doi:10.14581/jer.17003.

127 Margaret Gedde and Edward Maa, "Whole Cannabis Extract of High Concentration Cannabidiol May Calm Seizures in Highly Refractory Pediatric Epilepsies," *Realm of Caring*, Realm of Caring Foundation, March 2, 2016, https://www.theroc.us/gedde-study.

128 Shaun A. Hussain et al., "Perceived Efficacy of Cannabidiol-Enriched Cannabis Extracts for Treatment of Pediatric Epilepsy: A Potential Role for Infantile Spasms and Lennox–Gastaut Syndrome," *Epilepsy & Behavior* 47, (April 2015): 138–41, doi:10.1016/j.yebeh.2015.04.009.

129 Emma H. Kaplan et al., "Cannabidiol Treatment for Refractory Seizures in Sturge-Weber Syndrome," *Pediatric Neurology* 71, (June 2017): 18–23, doi:10.1016/j.pediatrneurol.2017.02.009.

130 Evan C. Rosenberg Pabitra H. Patra, and Benjamin J. Whalley, "Therapeutic Effects of Cannabinoids in Animal Models of Seizures,

Epilepsy, Epileptogenesis, and Epilepsy-Related Neuroprotection," *Epilepsy & Behavior* 70, Pt B (2017): 319–27, doi:10.1016/j.yebeh .2016.11.006.

131 Thomas W. Klein and Catherine A. Newton, "Therapeutic Potential of Cannabinoid-Based Drugs," *Advances in Experimental Medicine and Biology Immune-Mediated Diseases* 601 (2007): 395–413, doi:10.1007/978-0-387-72005-0_43.

132 M. Karsak et al., "Attenuation of Allergic Contact Dermatitis Through the Endocannabinoid System," *Science* 316, no. 5830 (2007): 1494–97, doi:10.1126/science.1142265.

133 Attila Oláh et al., "Cannabidiol Exerts Sebostatic and Anti-inflammatory Effects on Human Sebocytes," *Journal of Clinical Investigation* 124, no. 9 (2014): 3713–24, doi:10.1172/jci64628.

134 Ethan B. Russo, "Clinical Endocannabinoid Deficiency Reconsidered: Current Research Supports the Theory in Migraine, Fibromyalgia, Irritable Bowel, and Other Treatment-Resistant Syndromes," *Cannabis and Cannabinoid Research* 1, no. 1 (2016): 154–65, doi:10.1089/can.2016.0009.

135 Jonathan D. Wilkinson and Elizabeth M. Williamson, "Canna-binoids Inhibit Human Keratinocyte Proliferation through a Non-CB1/CB2 Mechanism and Have a Potential Therapeutic Value in the Treatment of Psoriasis," *Journal of Dermatological Science* 45, no. 2 (2006): 87–92, doi:10.1016/j.jdermsci.2006.10.009.

136 Daniel F. Kripke, "Hypnotic Drug Risks of Mortality, Infection, Depression, and Cancer: but Lack of Benefit," *F1000Research* 5, (May 2016): 918, doi:10.12688/f1000research.8729.1.

137 Ethan B. Russo, "Cannabidiol Claims and Misconceptions," *Trends in Pharmacological Sciences* 38, no. 3 (2017): 198–201, doi:10.1016/j.tips.2016.12.004.

138 Elisaldo A. Carlini and Jomar M. Cunha, "Hypnotic and Antiepileptic Effects of Cannabidiol," *The Journal of Clinical Pharmacology* 21, S1 (1981), doi:10.1002/j.1552-4604.1981.tb02622.x.

139   Atheer Zgair et al., "Dietary Fats and Pharmaceutical Lipid Excipients Increase Systemic Exposure to Orally Administered Cannabis and Cannabis-Based Medicines," *American Journal of Translational Research* 8, no. 8 (2016): 3448–59.

140   A. Hazekamp and J. T. Fischedick, "Cannabis—from Cultivar to Chemovar," *Drug Testing and Analysis* 4, no. 7–8 (2012): 660–67. doi:10.1002/dta.407.

141   G. C. Ceschel et al., "In Vitro Permeation through Porcine Buccal Mucosa of Salvia Desoleana Atzei & Picci Essential Oil from Topical Formulations," *International Journal of Pharmaceutics* 195, no. 1–2 (2000): 171–77, doi:10.1016/s0378-5173(99)00381-6.

142   Attila Olah et al., "Cannabidiol Exerts Sebostatic and Antiinflammatory Effects on Human Sebocytes," *Journal of Clinical Investigation* 124, no. 9 (2014): 3713–24, doi:10.1172/jci64628.

143   M. Jamontt et al., "The Effects of Δ9-Tetrahydrocannabinol and Cannabidiol Alone and in Combination on Damage, Inflammation Andin Vitromotility Disturbances in Rat Colitis," *British Journal of Pharmacology* 160, no. 3 (2010): 712–23, doi:10.1111/j.1476-5381.2010.00791.x.

144   Dustin Sulak, Russell Saneto, and Bonni Goldstein, "The Current Status of Artisanal Cannabis for the Treatment of Epilepsy in the United States," *Epilepsy & Behavior* 70, Pt B (2017): 328–33, doi:10.1016/j.yebeh.2016.12.032.

145   Deepak Cyril D'Souza et al., "Rapid Changes in Cannabinoid 1 Receptor Availability in Cannabis-Dependent Male Subjects After Abstinence From Cannabis," *Biological Psychiatry: Cognitive Neuroscience and Neuroimaging* 1, no. 1 (2016): 60–67, doi:10.1016/j.bpsc.2015.09.008.

Acknowledgments

This book would not be possible without the kind help and support of so many wonderful people!

First, we would like to thank the team at Ulysses Press for all the time, effort, and support they have given us in birthing *Healing with CBD*. Thanks to Casie Vogel, our lovely and talented editor who oversaw and supported us throughout, and thanks to Renee Rutledge for lending her keen eye for detail on copyediting. Thank you to Molly Conway for her public relations prowess, and the many other fine folks at Ulysses for all they have done behind the scenes.

Thank you to Andrea Burnett and her team at 4twenty Group for spreading the word and helping us connect to the folks who will find this book helpful in their healing journey.

We would like to thank Dr. Ethan Russo for his never-ending willingness to answer any and all questions. His generosity of mind and spirit went a long way in supporting the writing of this book.

We would also like to thank Eloise Theisen, AGPCNP-BC, a powerhouse of a nurse who takes the responsibility of educating and advocating for cannabis as seriously as Eileen does. Thank you, Eloise, for always answering the phone and sharing your wealth of knowledge and experience.

Special thanks to the American Cannabis Nurses Association (ACNA) for being a one-of-a-kind resource and platform to bring nurses into the field of cannabis medicine. It has provided the legitimacy needed to educate and help the patients they serve.

And finally, we would not be here without the thousands of patients, advocates, and educators who have shaped both Eileen's and Lauren's journey, but more importantly the ever-changing and constantly growing cannabis landscape.

Thank you!

About the Authors

Eileen Konieczny, RN, has spent decades working to alleviate the suffering of those she cared for as a bedside registered nurse who specialized in cancer. Since 2008, after learning how safe and therapeutic the cannabis plant can be, Eileen stepped out of her comfort zone and began advocating on behalf of its use as medicine.

International Nurse Leader, President, Strategist, and Cannabis Nurse are all titles that Eileen holds from her work and knowledge around cannabis. She has educated thousands on the benefits of cannabis and played an instrumental role in securing safe access to medical cannabis for 23 million people.

Eileen lives in New York's Hudson Valley with her family, pets, and farm animals. Eggs are for sale when the hens are laying.

Lauren Wilson is a professional food lover. After graduating from Toronto's George Brown Chef School in 2008, she followed a trail of crumbs to Brooklyn, New York, where she has been writing cookbooks, teaching cooking classes, and working in the restaurant scene happily. She is the author of the *The Walking Dead: The Official Cookbook and Survival Guide* and *The Art of Eating Through the Zombie Apocalypse: A Cookbook and Culinary Survival Guide.*

Lauren is also a professional cannabis lover. She initially came to the cannabis world as a recreational user in her youth, and has since developed a far more deep and meaningful relationship to the plant as a patient seeking a natural and nontoxic option for chronic pain relief. It was through this newfound relationship that Lauren came to understand the current legal, political, and social landscape surrounding cannabis. She has since connected to Eileen Konieczny and many others in the passionate community working tirelessly to make this sacred plant accessible to any and all who could benefit from it. As coauthor of *Healing with CBD*, Lauren hopes to help and support those who may not have considered cannabis therapeutics, offering the knowledge and confidence they might need to try it.